CW00846934

MCQs FOR THE DRCOG

Dedicated to Sue, Carrie, Lisa, Richard, Ellie, Edward and Mr Alan Sugar of Amstrad Computers without whose help. . . .

For Churchill Livingstone

Publisher: Peter Richardson
Editorial co-ordination: Editorial Resources Unit
Production Controller: Neil Dickson
Design: Design Resources Unit
Sales Promotion Executive: Louise Johnstone

MCQs for the DRCOG

Matthew Hoghton
MB ChB MRCP(UK) DRCOG FPcert MRCGP
General Practitioner, Bristol

Patrick Hogston
MB BS BSc LRCP FRCS MRCOG
Consultant Obstetrician and Gynaecologist,
St Mary's Hospital, Portsmouth
Clinical Teacher, University of Southampton,
Southampton

Foreword by
Gordon M. Stirrat
MA MD FRCOG
Professor of Obstetrics and Gynaecology,
University of Bristol, Bristol

CHURCHILL LIVINGSTONE
EDINBURGH LONDON MELBOURNE NEW YORK AND TOKYO 1991

CHURCHILL LIVINGSTONE
Medical Division of Longman Group UK Limited

Distributed in the United States of America by
Churchill Livingstone Inc., 1560 Broadway, New York,
N.Y. 10036, and by associated companies, branches
and representatives throughout the world.

First published 1991
  Reprinted 1994

ISBN 0-443-04469-4

British Library Cataloguing in Publication Data

Hoghton, Matthew
  MCQs for the DRCOG.
  1. Gynaecology. Obstetrics
  I. Title II. Hogston, Patrick
  618

Library of Congress Cataloging in Publication Data

Hoghton, Matthew
    MCQs for the DRCOG/Matthew Hoghton, Patrick Hogston; foreword
by Gordon M. Stirrat.
      p.   cm.
    Includes index.
    ISBN 0-443-04469-4
    1. Gynecology—Examinations, questions, etc. 2. Obstetrics—
Examinations, questions, etc. I. Hogston, Patrick. II. Title.
    [DNLM: 1. Gynecology—examination questions. 2. Obstetrics—
examination questions. WQ 18 H716m]
RG111.H58 1991
618'.076—dc20
DNLM/DLC
for Library of Congress   90–15130

The
publisher's
policy is to use
paper manufactured
from sustainable forests

Printed and bound in Great Britain by
Butler & Tanner Ltd, Frome and London

Foreword

If, as we are told, confession is good for the soul I should feel better after writing this foreword. The fact of the matter is that I dislike MCQs. No, let me be more accurate – I *detest* them. Why do I feel so strongly about this widely used form of assessment? My first reason is that the structure of the questions often requires definite decisions about variable and indefinite issues. Second, this form of examination was being introduced experimentally when I was a student and I do not think I passed any of them!

I suspect that my feelings towards MCQs are shared by a great many but there is no doubt that as a form of assessment MCQs are here to stay and we have to accommodate to them. That is why this excellent book by Matthew Hoghton and Patrick Hogston is so welcome for candidates for the DRCOG.

Having accepted the invitation to write this foreword I felt that I had to put myself to the test. I therefore 'sat the exam.' You will be pleased to hear that I passed (although I did mark it myself). My mark must remain secret because I did not gain 90 let alone 100%! My errors fell into the following categories: (1) I didn't know and guessed (fatal!) (2) I thought I knew and was wrong (OK, so no-one's perfect!) (3) I misread the stem (stupid) and (4) I disagreed with the given answer (a professor's prerogative!).

Can I therefore reinforce the instructions given to you by the authors at the beginning of the book. The technique for MCQs is different, and can be practised and improved upon. Having answered the questions in this book once, review your marks and repeat the process until you begin to be satisfied with your performance (and then do it again). You will not only be more proficient at the technique but will have learned a great deal about the topics.

Let me therefore finally commend this book strongly to you as of great potential value for those sitting the DRCOG, I'm sorry I can't write any more – I have to take the exam again!

Gordon M. Stirrat

Preface

Since January 1990, the Diploma Examination of the Royal College of Obstetricians and Gynaecologists (DRCOG) has introduced Multiple Choice Questions into the written paper. Most candidates will have little opportunity to practise MCQ questions and hence the need for this book.

The aim of these practice examinations is to allow candidates to assess their knowledge under exam conditions. The answers are given at the end of each examination along with an explanation and further information where relevant. An index is included which will help the candidate to ensure he/she has covered the important topics. We have also provided a small list of recommended books.

M.H.
P.H.

Acknowledgements

We are grateful to Chrissy Austin and Peter Richardson of Churchill Livingstone for supporting us in this endeavour. We are also grateful to the following contributors: Dr S. J. Armstrong MRCP, FRCR, Senior Registrar in Radiology, South Western Region; Dr P. Curtis MRCOG, Research Registrar in Obstetrics and Gynaecology, Royal Free Hospital, London; and Dr S. Whitcroft MRCOG, Research Registrar in Obstetrics and Gynaecology, King's College Hospital, London.

Contents

Instructions for the MCQ Paper in Obstetrics and Gynaecology for DRCOG

The paper consists of 40 five-part multiple choice questions. The time allowed for completion of the MCQ examination is 1 hour 15 minutes. The answer sheet is marked by computer and must be completed in HB pencil only. Each lozenge of the answer sheet should be filled with a bold dark line; a faint line is not read by the computer. A rubber is provided.

Each question consists of an initial statement followed by five items identified by the letters a, b, c, d and e. The answer sheet contains a row of five boxes for each question labelled accordingly. In each box there are three lozenges labelled T for true, F for false and DK for don't know. If you know a particular item of a question to be true or false, black out either the true (T) or the false (F) lozenge. If you do not know the answer you must black out the don't know (DK) lozenge.

SPECIMEN QUESTION AND ANSWERS

During breast feeding
a Mastitis may be resolved by continued breast feeding
b Superficial mastitis should be treated with antibiotics
c Twins will require supplementary bottle feeding
d Lactating women should drink extra fluids
e Demand feeding produces obese babies

Answers **a** and **b** are TRUE, **c**, **d** and **e** are FALSE

Your answer sheet to this question would look like this when correctly filled in:

	A		B		C		D		E
T	⬤	T	⬤	T	◯	T	◯	T	◯
F	◯	F	◯	F	⬤	F	⬤	F	⬤
DK	◯	DK	◯	DK	◯	DK	◯	DK	◯

T means TRUE, F means FALSE, DK means DON'T KNOW

If you know the answer to **a**, **b**, **c** and **d** but do not know the answer to **e** then your answer sheet will be completed as follows:

A	B	C	D	E
T ⬤	T ⬤	T ◯	T ◯	T ◯
F ◯	F ◯	F ⬤	F ⬤	F ◯
DK ◯	DK ◯	DK ◯	DK ◯	DK ⬤

Each item correctly answered (i.e. a true statement indicated as true or a false statement indicated as false) is awarded one mark (+1). For each incorrect answer, one mark is deducted (−1). For those items marked don't know, no marks are awarded or deducted (0).

The completed question book will be collected at the end of the time allowed for the MCQ examination. The essay paper will then be issued. It is not possible to leave the examination hall between completion of the MCQ paper and the start of the essay paper.

General Advice for Taking MCQ Examinations

PREPARATION FOR TAKING EXAMINATIONS

1. Do plenty of MCQs.
2. Talk about Obstetrics and Gynaecology with your colleagues.
3. Ask for teaching from senior colleagues and attend lectures at every opportunity. Try to get involved in the discussions.
4. Practise techniques, e.g. essay plans, vivas.
5. Try to take regular exercise between periods of study.
6. Avoid too many stimulants, especially coffee (take up decaffeinated!).
7. Go to bed at a regular time.
8. Plan your available time to cover the subject matter, rather than spending too much time on detail.

ANSWERING MCQs

1. Read the instructions carefully.
2. Fill in your name and candidate number.
3. Plan your time.
4. Allow at least 15 minutes for transcribing your answers on to the answer sheet.
5. You are unlikely to know definitely all the answers. If you have no knowledge about a particular subject, do not guess, but if you feel that you are more than 50% certain of the answer you should probably attempt it.
6. Mark your responses in the appropriate box.

INTERPRETATION OF TERMS

Maybe — unlikely to be false
Always — likely to be false
Usually — over 60% occurrence
Characteristic — if absent, the diagnosis is unlikely
Rarely — less than 10%
Majority — greater than 50%
Can occur — if it has occurred once, it can occur again

AFTER THE EXAMINATION

1. Remember that an exam is only an exam; failing it is not the end of the world. Many excellent senior doctors have retaken postgraduate exams.
2. Go and relax. Avoid post-mortems, especially with people anxious to discuss how well they did. Also avoid having to support and reassure others.
3. Don't belittle yourself.
4. Apart from pride, all you lose is money.
5. Look after your loved ones, remember they are taking the exam with you.

1. Paper A

A1 **Blood pressure in pregnancy:**
- **a** Rises gradually from the first trimester until delivery
- **b** Should be measured using a large cuff if the upper arm circumference is greater than 35 cm
- **c** Will be artificially lowered if taken with the patient lying
- **d** Will show at least one reading of 140/90 mmHg in 20% of women
- **e** Phase V of Korotkoff's sound is used in the measurement of diastolic pressure

A2 **Pre-eclampsia:**
- **a** Is commoner in women with a previous miscarriage
- **b** May present with abdominal pain and vomiting
- **c** Is commoner in smokers than in non-smokers
- **d** Is a common cause of symmetrical intra-uterine growth retardation
- **e** Can be treated with diuretics in early cases

A3 **The following conditions can be diagnosed by high resolution ultrasound at 20 weeks of pregnancy:**
- **a** Holoprosencephaly
- **b** Gastroschisis
- **c** Cystic fibrosis
- **d** Urethral valves
- **e** Hypoplastic left heart

A4 **A pregnant woman with asthma:**
- **a** Should not be treated with aminophylline
- **b** Can be safely treated with steroids
- **c** Is more vulnerable to 'status asthmaticus' in labour
- **d** Has at least twice the chance of having a child who will develop asthma than does a non-asthmatic woman
- **e** Should avoid beta-sympathomimetic drugs

A5   Thromboembolic disease in pregnancy:
   a   Is a major cause of maternal death
   b   Should be treated with coumarins in the first trimester
   c   Venography and isotope lung scanning must not be used
   d   Preventative treatment with subcutaneous heparin has no risk to the mother
   e   Is commoner in women after caesarean section

A6   The following are compatible with a normal outcome of pregnancy:
   a   Blood pressure at booking of 140/100 mmHg
   b   Weight gain throughout pregnancy of 2 kg
   c   Severe lower limb oedema
   d   Blood urea of 12 mmol/l
   e   Thalassaemia major

A7   In pregnancy:
   a   A haemoglobin of 11 g/dl is the lower limit of normal according to WHO guidelines
   b   A low serum iron with a low total iron binding capacity suggests iron deficiency
   c   The overall total iron requirement is approximately 1000 mg
   d   Iron absorption is increased
   e   The plasma volume rises by about 1200 ml

A8   The following statements about the neonate are true:
   a   An Apgar score of 3 at 5 minutes predicts a 50% chance of subsequent cerebral palsy
   b   Continuous electronic fetal heart rate monitoring in labour reduces the incidence of cerebral palsy
   c   Poor feeding and jaundice may be the only signs of neonatal septicaemia
   d   The commonest cause of death in the first year of life is the sudden infant death syndrome (SIDS)
   e   Ophthalmia neonatorum is a notifiable disease

A9   The following conditions have an autosomal recessive mode of inheritance:
   a   Achondroplasia
   b   Phenylketonuria
   c   Tuberous sclerosis
   d   Huntingdon's chorea
   e   Retinitis pigmentosa

A10   The following are risk factors for shoulder dystocia:
   a   Maternal weight of 110 kg
   b   Rotational forceps delivery
   c   Gestational diabetes
   d   42 weeks gestation
   e   Oxytocin augmentation for primary dysfunctional labour

A11 Which of the following increase the risk of a caesarean section in a primigravida at 41 weeks gestation?:
  a Fresh meconium liquor seen in labour
  b Induction of labour for prolonged rupture of the membranes
  c Continuous electronic fetal monitoring
  d Oxytocin augmentation for secondary arrest at 8 cm
  e Artificial rupture of membranes as part of active management of labour

A12 Primary postpartum haemorrhage (PPH):
  a Is reduced by active management of the third stage of labour
  b Is usually caused by trauma to the genital tract
  c Is less common in multiparous women
  d Is more common in women who experienced it in previous pregnancies
  e When the cause of maternal death is often due to delay in performing hysterectomy

A13 Carcinoma of the cervix:
  a Kills more women than carcinoma of the ovary
  b Is more common in social class V
  c May be related to the sexual behaviour of the woman's partner
  d Would kill fewer women if there was a national screening programme for all women over 35
  e Can be present with a normal cervical smear

A14 Ectopic pregnancy:
  a Has a higher incidence in women with copper intra-uterine contraceptive devices (IUCDs) than sexually active women not using contraception
  b Is excluded by the presence of an intra-uterine gestational sac on ultrasound
  c Reduces the chance of the woman having a live child
  d Is excluded by a negative serum beta HCG
  e Accounts for 20% of pregnancies occurring after failed sterilisation

A15 The combined oral contraceptive pill:
  a Is relatively safe to continue up to the age of 40 in a woman who does not smoke
  b Alters glucose tolerance
  c Increases the incidence of vaginal candidiasis
  d May be used as a means of postcoital contraception
  e Increases the risk of ovarian cancer

A16 Hormone replacement therapy for postmenopausal women:
a Has similar risks to the combined oral contraceptive pill
b Reduces the incidence of fractures of the vertebral bodies
c Should be given as oestrogen-only in women post hysterectomy
d May increase the risk of breast cancer
e May reduce mortality from cardiovascular disease

A17 Intra-uterine contraceptive devices:
a Should not be inserted immediately after menstruation, as the device will be expelled
b Should be removed at the menopause
c Can be used 4 days after unprotected intercourse to prevent implantation
d Should be removed if possible if pregnancy occurs
e Cause more pelvic infection in nulliparous women than in parous women

A18 A woman who complains of menorrhagia:
a May be losing a normal amount of blood per month
b Can be successfully treated with non-steroidal anti-inflammatory drugs
c Is unlikely to be under 40 years of age
d Will be helped by a D&C in most cases
e Should be referred, if she is over 40 years of age, to a gynaecologist

A19 A couple complain of inability to conceive after two years of unprotected intercourse:
a The cause is more likely to be in the female partner
b Ovulation can be confirmed by estimating the Day 21 progesterone
c Are more likely to be over 35 years of age
d If a spontaneous pregnancy ensues, the likelihood of its being ectopic is greater than in the general population
e The cause could be Salazopyrin therapy in the male partner

A20 Endometriosis:
a Is associated with low parity
b Is worsened by intra-uterine contraceptive devices (IUCDs)
c Is a rare cause of haematuria
d Can be treated with continuous use of the combined oral contraceptive pill
e If the ovaries are surgically removed at 35 years of age, oestrogen replacement should be given

A21 Spontaneous abortion at 8 weeks:
    a Is uncommon once a live fetus has been seen on ultrasound
    b Is often due to chromosomal abnormalities in the conceptus
    c Can be prevented by injections of hCG
    d Should be treated with anti-D in Rhesus-negative women
    e May lead to acute pelvic inflammatory disease

A22 At the climacteric:
    a The sensation of hot flushes is due to stimulation of the temperature regulation centre
    b The incidence of fractures starts to increase
    c Plasma cholesterol and triglyceride levels fall
    d Oestrogen therapy by vaginal cream does not result in endometrial hyperplasia
    e Hormone replacement therapy (HRT) increases the risk of thromboembolism

A23 Ovarian cancer:
    a May present with dyspepsia
    b Is commoner in social class V
    c Usually presents as stage I or II disease
    d Kills more women than all other gynaecological cancers
    e Is more common in previous users of the combined oral contraceptive pill

A24 Secondary amenorrhoea:
    a Is more common in athletes and ballet dancers
    b Often follows cessation of the oral contraceptive pill for at least 6 months
    c May follow dilatation and curettage
    d May lead to osteoporosis
    e Due to ovarian failure, will cause a low serum FSH/LH ratio

A25 Pre-term delivery:
    a The risk is increased by smoking
    b Is more likely after a previous first trimester termination
    c Is less likely in diabetic women
    d Can be prevented by cervical cerclage in most cases
    e Occurs in approximately 15% of women admitted with painful contractions before 37 weeks

A26 Therapy with beta-sympathomimetic drugs to treat pre-term labour:
    a Improves the outcome for the baby
    b The drugs cross the placenta
    c Can cause fatal pulmonary oedema
    d Is contra-indicated in asthmatics
    e Can cause hyperglycaemic ketoacidosis

A27 Antenatal care should include:
  a Serial vaginal examination when there is a previous history of termination of pregnancy
  b Testing for hepatitis B in women from Vietnam
  c Haemoglobin electrophoresis in women from Pakistan
  d Routine use of kick charts to prevent intra-uterine death
  e Iron and folic acid supplements given to women with twins

A28 Human immunodeficiency virus (HIV) infection:
  a Is associated with an increased risk of pre-term delivery
  b Causes characteristic fetal abnormalities
  c Can be transmitted in the breast milk
  d Can cause maternal meningitis
  e Is associated with squamous cell carcinoma of the rectum

A29 The following are more common in the male child:
  a Talipes equinovarus
  b Congenital dislocation of the hip
  c Pyloric stenosis
  d Isolated cleft palate
  e Hirchsprung's disease

A30 Physiological neonatal jaundice:
  a May occur on the first day after birth
  b Will require phototherapy if the bilirubin rises to 200 μmol/l
  c Will cause a positive Coombs' test
  d Is better treated by bottle feeding
  e Is more common in pre-term babies

A31 The pre-menstrual syndrome:
  a Is relieved by hysterectomy
  b Is relieved by a sympathetic doctor
  c Can be treated with spironolactone
  d Lasts throughout the menstrual cycle
  e Occurs while on the oral contraceptive pill

A32 Depoprovera (medroxyprogesterone acetate):
  a Eventually causes amenorrhoea
  b Cannot be given to women with sickle cell anaemia
  c Is as effective as the combined oral contraceptive pill
  d Can be given to lactating women
  e Causes weight gain

A33 The following may be diagnosed by chorionic villus biopsy:
  a Alpha thalassaemia
  b Cystic fibrosis
  c Haemophilia
  d Edward's syndrome (trisomy 18)
  e Fragile X syndrome

A34 A woman with a raised serum alpha fetoprotein (AFP) at 16 weeks:
- a Has a 50% chance of carrying a fetus with spina bifida
- b Is more significant if the woman is an insulin-dependent diabetic
- c Has an increased risk of a child with Down's syndrome
- d Should have a detailed ultrasound
- e May have an intra-uterine death

A35 Breech presentation:
- a Occurs in 2% of all labours at term
- b May be due to an abnormal fetus
- c Increases the risk of prolapse of the cord
- d Increases the risk of postpartum haemorrhage (PPH)
- e Causes an increased perinatal mortality due to asphyxia

A36 Which of the following are true of the social security benefits for pregnant women in the United Kingdom?:
- a A pregnant woman, who is entitled to Statutory Maternal Pay (SMP) should inform her employers 7 days before she intends to stop work
- b The form Mat B1(A) can be issued by the GP or midwife from 20 weeks
- c If a woman is not eligible for SMP, she may be entitled to the maternity allowance
- d If a woman claims maternity allowance after confinement, she should use form Mat B1(B)
- e Dental treatment is free for mothers up to 1 year after the baby is born

A37 Acute pelvic inflammatory disease (PID):
- a Is most commonly due to gonococcus in the UK
- b Can only be diagnosed accurately by laparoscopy
- c Gives a 10–20% chance of infertility after one attack
- d May follow spontaneous miscarriage
- e Requires tetracycline as part of treatment

A38 Gestational diabetes mellitus:
- a Will require insulin therapy if ketonuria develops on diet treatment
- b Is accurately screened for by urine testing for glucose
- c Can be screened for by serum fructosamine
- d Is diagnosed by a 100 g oral glucose tolerance test in the UK
- e Is more common in siblings of diabetics

A39 Breastfeeding:
- a Should be carried out every 4 hours
- b Should be stopped if mastitis occurs
- c Requires extra fluid intake for the mother
- d Should not start until 4 hours after delivery
- e Usually fails due to poor advice and lack of encouragement

A40 Bleeding at 4 weeks post delivery:
  a May be physiological
  b Is exacerbated by the progestogen-only pill
  c Is best treated by D&C
  d May be due to choriocarcinoma
  e May be due to carcinoma of the cervix

2. Paper A Answers

A1 a False
Blood pressure falls in the second trimester, then rises in the third trimester.

b True
A standard cuff (12×23 cm) will not encompass the arm of 5% of hypertensive pregnant patients. A large cuff must be used to avoid overdiagnosing hypertension in obese women.

c True
This position may cause supine hypotension, as the gravid uterus can impair venous return via the inferior vena cava. A semi-recumbent position with lateral tilt and with the cuff at the same level as the heart will produce more accurate results.

d True
This is true predominantly for the second half of pregnancy. Only 2% of women will have a reading this high in the first half of pregnancy.

e False
In some pregnant women, the Korotkoff V phase can be heard at zero cuff pressure. For this reason, Korotkoff IV phase should be taken as the diastolic reading in pregnant women.

A2 a False
Underweight primigravida are particularly affected. Other risk factors for pre-eclampsia include: a family history of pre-eclampsia, age under 20 or over 35, chronic hypertension and renal disease.

b True
The presence of these symptoms suggest that the woman is seriously ill with impending eclampsia.

c False
Smokers have a lower incidence of pre-eclampsia than non-smokers. However, smoking is associated with other adverse obstetric outcomes, e.g. low-birthweight babies.

d False
It causes asymmetrical growth retardation.

e False
Vasodilator drugs, such as nifedipine and hydralazine, may be used in the treatment of severe pre-eclampsia. Other useful anti-hypertensive drugs include methyldopa and the beta blockers. Diuretics are reserved for the treatment of heart failure.

A3   a True
This abnormality in its most severe form leads to a single ventricle within the cranium, and is associated with midline facial abnormalities. There is always absence of the falx cerebri, which distinguishes it from *hydrancephaly*, in which the cranium is fluid-filled and brain tissue is absent.

b True
Gastroschisis is a defect in the anterior abdominal wall. There is normal insertion of the umbilical cord, the hernia occurring usually to the right of the midline. The contents of the hernia have no covering membrane, as opposed to an *omphalocoele* which occurs through the umbilicus in the midline. The presence of an omphalocoele is associated with other midline abnormalities, and 50% have cardiac and chromosomal abnormalities. In both conditions, serum alpha fetoprotein is raised.

c False
No anatomical markers exist for cystic fibrosis. It can now be diagnosed in some families by chorionic villus biopsy.

d True
Posterior urethral valves occur almost exclusively in male infants, and cause varying degrees of dilatation of the urinary tract. Approximately 25% of affected fetuses will have a chromosome abnormality, and termination may be considered.

e True
The early diagnosis of cardiac lesions ensures delivery in a specialist centre where treatable conditions can be dealt with urgently. Hypoplastic left heart is a fatal abnormality.

A4   a False
Aminophylline has been used in pregnancy with no adverse effects on the fetus. It is important not to undertreat asthma or any other medical condition in pregnancy.

b True
There is some risk of fetal growth retardation with regular steroid therapy in excess of 12 mg/day. It is unclear whether the cause of this growth retardation is arterial hypoxaemia or steroid therapy in pregnant women with severe asthma.

c False
Status asthmaticus is uncommon during labour, and is thought to be protected against by high levels of endogenous catecholamines and corticosteroids.

d True
The inheritance is polygenic.

e False
Beta-sympathomimetic drugs, such as salbutamol, are safe for the fetus. They may cause maternal pulmonary oedema if given intravenously, but are safe if inhaled. They are used in the treatment of premature labour in non-asthmatics, but they do not seem to delay the onset of labour nor prolong labour in women with asthma.

A5 a True
The last confidential enquiry into maternal deaths in England and Wales lists pulmonary embolism and hypertension as the most frequent causes of maternal death, at 10 per 1 million pregnancies. The incidence of pulmonary embolism is 5 times greater in pregnant than in non-pregnant women, the most dangerous period being the first 7 days of the puerperium.

b False
Warfarin (a coumarin derivative) is teratogenic. The effects on the fetus include saddle nose, frontal bossing, midface hypoplasia, short stature, cardiac defects, mental retardation and blindness. Warfarin should be avoided in the first trimester and around the time of delivery. Patients with thrombosis and thromboembolism in pregnancy should be treated with intravenous heparin for 5–7 days, followed by intermittent subcutaneous heparin or warfarin depending on gestation.

c False
25–50% of patients with suspected venous thrombosis do not have thrombosis, therefore it is important to weigh the risks of unnecessary anticoagulation against the small potential risk of radiation. If venography is thought to be necessary, a lead apron shielding the pelvis gives protection to the fetus.

d False
Local bruising, thrombocytopenia, over-anticoagulation, hypersensitivity reactions and bone demineralisation (osteoporosis) may all occur with subcutaneous heparin.

e True
The risk of fatal pulmonary embolism is 10 times greater after caesarean section than after vaginal delivery. Other factors found to be important by the confidential enquiries include: age, parity, excessive obesity, hospitalisation and restricted activity (especially if for an obstetric complication). Suppression of lactation by oestrogen, a history of previous DVT or PE, the presence of lupus anticoagulant and hereditary thrombotic disease are also risk factors.

A6 a True
The outcome relates to developing superimposed pre-eclampsia, but it is probably advisable to treat this level of hypertension for maternal reasons.

b True
Weight gain is a poor predictor of outcome, and low weight is compatible with a normal-sized infant. The average weight gain in pregnancy is 10–12 kg, but many feel routine weighing in pregnancy could be abandoned.

c True
This is usually physiological due to fluid retention and, to a lesser degree, obstruction from the gravid uterus.

d False
Chronic renal failure has a poor outcome and most women will never become pregnant.

e False
Few survive to childbearing age anyway, although modern therapy with iron-chelating agents does prolong survival.

A7 a True
The mean minimum value accepted by the World Health Organisation is 11.0 g/dl (at sea-level). For non-pregnant women, it is 12.0 g/dl. In the UK, haemoglobin levels below 10 g/dl in the second and third trimesters are likely to be abnormal and should be investigated.

b False
In iron deficiency anaemia, there is a low serum iron and raised total iron binding capacity (TIBC), with a hypochromic microcytic film and a low serum ferritin. Chronic disorders, such as SLE and rheumatoid arthritis, produce an anaemia with a low serum iron and TIBC.

c True
The increase in maternal red cell mass requires a net gain of 500–600 mg during pregnancy. 250–300 mg is also required for transfer to the fetus. The daily requirement is 3–4 times that of a non-pregnant woman.

d True
The increased demand for iron is met by increasing the absorption of iron from the gut and by mobilisation of maternal stores.

e True
The normal plasma volume of a non-pregnant woman is 2600 ml and increases in singleton pregnancies by 1250 ml. Most of the increase in volume occurs before 32 weeks of gestation. This increase is related to birthweight, and is greater in multiple pregnancy and in second and subsequent pregnancies.

A8 a False
While a low Apgar score of 3 at 5 minutes post delivery is associated with an increased incidence of cerebral palsy, only 16% of those that survive have cerebral palsy. If the score is still 3 at 20 minutes, 57% will have cerebral palsy. However, it should be remembered that 75% of children with cerebral palsy have 5-minute Apgar scores of 7 or greater, and the strongest correlation with subsequent cerebral palsy is low birthweight (22 times more likely in infants below 1500 g compared to those over 2500 g).

b False
Electronic fetal monitoring measures fetal asphyxia, but is a poor predictor of subsequent cerebral palsy. This may be because cerebral palsy may not be a consequence of perinatal asphyxia.

c True
Other signs include: a rise or fall in temperature, drowsiness, vomiting, failure to gain weight, an anxious look and a greyish pallor of the skin. The commonest causative organisms are *E. coli*, *Staphylococcus*, *Pseudomonas aeruginosa*, *Proteus* and *Haemolytic streptococcus*.

d True
One in 500 infants will die suddenly and unexpectedly. The risk factors include: low birthweight, twin pregnancy, bottle-feeding, young mothers, illegitimacy, poor housing conditions, excessive cot covers and a prone sleeping position.

e True
It is notifiable in the UK except in Northern Ireland.

A9 a False
Autosomal dominant. Other examples of autosomal dominant disorders include: facioscapulohumeral dystrophy, Gilbert's syndrome, Marfan's syndrome, neurofibromatosis, osteogenesis imperfecta tarda, polycystic disease of the kidney (adult form), tuberous sclerosis and Von Willebrand's disease.

b True
Enzyme defects tend to be autosomal recessive. Other examples include: albinism, congenital adrenal hyperplasia, cystic fibrosis, galactosaemia, Gaucher's disease, glycogen storage diseases, Tay-Sachs disease and Wilson's disease.

c False
Tuberous sclerosis is inherited as an autosomal dominant. Clinical features include: adenoma sebaceum, subungual fibromas, shagreen patches and cafe-au-lait spots. Hamartomas, intracranial gliomas, cardiac rhabdomyomas and interstitial lung disease are also seen.

d False
Huntingdon's chorea is inherited as an autosomal dominant, and usually presents after the age of 30. It causes choreiform movements associated with progressive dementia.

e True
Retinitis pigmentosa causes progressive blindness from an early age, and most types are autosomal recessive. Autosomal dominant and X-linked recessive types do occur.

A10 a True
Shoulder dystocia is a very serious and often totally unexpected complication of the second stage of labour. All personnel involved in intrapartum care must be able to recognise shoulder dystocia and take appropriate action. Big women have big babies, although the size of the fetus may be masked by the size of the mother.

b True
Mid-cavity forceps is a risk factor, because it may represent some degree of disproportion as the fetal head has failed to pass the pelvic outlet.

c True
Any condition leading to macrosomia increases the risk of shoulder dystocia (see **a**). In diabetics, the fetal head may be of normal size but the body is disproportionately large and the shoulders fail to enter the pelvis as the head is delivering.

d True
The mean birthweight at 42 weeks is greater than at 40 weeks. Almost all the growth will have occurred by 40 weeks, and so it should not be deduced that elective delivery at 40 weeks would solve the problem.

e False
Dysfunctional labour is due to poor uterine action. Secondary arrest of labour, particularly if response to oxytocin is poor, may indicate relative disproportion.

A11 a True
Although it need not mean the baby is distressed.

b True
Any induction increases the risk of caesarean section.

c True
Although with fetal blood sampling this can be reduced.

d True
This suggests disproportion or OP position.

e False
Cord prolapse is no more common than after spontaneous rupture.

A12 a True
Primary postpartum haemorrhage (PPH) is defined as blood loss of more than 500 ml from the genital tract in the first 24 hours after delivery. An oxytocic given with delivery of the anterior shoulder, followed by controlled cord traction to deliver the placenta, will reduce the incidence of PPH.

b False
Uterine atony is the commonest cause of PPH (90%). Trauma accounts for 7%, and coagulation defects for the remaining 3%.

c False
Grand multiparity (4 or more births) predisposes to postpartum haemorrhage. One reason may be an increasing amount of fibrous tissue within the uterine wall hindering effective contraction of the uterus.

d True
These women should be booked for consultant delivery. Other factors predisposing to PPH include: uterine over-distension (e.g. polyhydramnios, multiple pregnancy), multiparity, antepartum haemorrhage and poor uterine action.

e True
Delay in performing hysterectomy for PPH is a recurrent theme in the confidential enquiries into maternal death.

A13 a False
There are about 2000 deaths due to cervical cancer annually in England and Wales (3% of cancer deaths in women). The average GP will see one new case every 5 years. Ovarian cancer kills twice as many women as cervical cancer, about 4000 deaths annually in England and Wales.

b True
Cervical cancer is 5 times more common in social class V than it is in the professional classes. It is more common in urban than in rural areas.

c True
The number of sexual contacts of a woman's partner has been found to be a significant risk factor in the development of cervical cancer. Othe risk factors include age of woman at first intercourse, a large number of sexual partners and lower socioeconomic group. The relationship with the human papilloma viruses is unclear, and there is no relationship with herpes virus type II. The relationship of cervical cancer to parity is unclear.

d True
There is no national screening programme in the UK.

e True
It has been estimated that there may be a 10% false-negative rate. Necrotic tumours may result in negative cytology.

A14 a False
Many sources suggest that use of the IUCD increases the risk of ectopic pregnancy. Any form of contraception reduces the incidence of pregnancy, and therefore of ectopic pregnancy. Permanent users of the IUCD have the same risk of ectopic pregnancy as those who have never used them, except with the no longer used Progestasert (a progesterone releasing IUCD) which did increase the incidence of ectopics. However, if pregnancy does occur in a woman using an IUCD, the relative risk of an ectopic pregnancy is considerably increased. Pill users are at least risk (one-third the incidence with IUCDs). The aetiological factors identified for ectopic pregnancy are: pelvic inflammatory disease, increasing age, race (commoner in non-whites), previous tubal surgery or in vitro fertilisation (IVF), and a previous ectopic pregnancy.

b False
The figure given in textbooks for the likelihood of an intra-uterine gestation and an ectopic pregnancy occurring simultaneously is 1 in 30 000. However, with an increasing prevalence of pelvic inflammatory disease and induced ovulation, recent American studies suggest the incidence is significantly higher, 1 in 7000. A 'pseudo-gestational sac' may be seen within the uterus in an ectopic pregnancy due to ectopic hormonal stimulation of the endometrium. This is seen in 10–20% of ectopic pregnancies on ultrasound scanning.

c True
Only one-third of women with previous ectopics who wish to conceive will produce a live infant, and 10% will have another ectopic pregnancy.

d True
Sensitive assays are now available which can always exclude early pregnancy. Older types of pregnancy testing involving agglutination techniques were less sensitive and so could be negative in the presence of an ectopic pregnancy.

e True
These women tend to present late. Sterilisation should not be performed if the woman has had unprotected intercourse in the preceding 2 weeks.

A15 a True
The vascular effects of the contraceptive pill are closely linked with cigarette smoking.

b True
Although of minimal importance for healthy women. If they are used for diabetics, then careful review of their insulin requirements will be required.

c False
Recent evidence is against this, and it appears equally as common in users of barrier contraception.

d True
The oral contraceptive pill can be used for postcoital contraception within 72 hours of intercourse. Two 50 µg pills 12 hours apart will cause a withdrawal bleed within 21 days in 98% of women. It is important to confirm that this has occurred.

e False
It is highly protective against ovarian cancer, and this protection increases with use. The mechanism probably lies in the suppression of ovarian function.

A16 a False
The equivalent amounts of oestrogen and progestogen in HRT are significantly less than those necessary in the combined pill in order to suppress ovulation. Consequently, the incidence of side-effects is less with HRT. Hormone replacement therapy does not lower the very high FSH and LH levels found in postmenopausal women to any degree.

b True
The expected fracture rate of 40 fractures/1000 patient years is significantly reduced to only 3 fractures/1000 patient years, even in osteoporotic postmenopausal women.

c True
Progestogens are given to women who have not had a hysterectomy. It protects against the risk of endometrial carcinoma, which is increased with unopposed oestrogens. However, progestogens may possibly reverse the beneficial effects of oestrogens on plasma lipids and lipoproteins.

d True
A potential carcinogenic effect of HRT on the breast (which is known to be an oestrogen target organ) has not yet been proved. However, pre-existing breast cancer is an absolute contraindication to hormone replacement therapy. Other absolute contraindications include hormone-dependent cancers of the endometrium and ovary. Relative contraindications are: pre-existing hypertension, a history of thromboembolic disease, myocardial infarction, benign breast disease, diabetes, fibroids, gallbladder disease and familial hyperlipidaemia. It would seem sensible for GPs to ask specialists about women with these relative contraindications who have severe menopausal symptoms.

e True
Oestrogens have a beneficial effect on the incidence of ischaemic heart disease in postmenopausal women, as compared to the adverse effect of oestrogens given in the combined oral contraceptive pill. This beneficial effect also applies to women who smoke. Progestogens are associated with an increased incidence of ischaemic heart disease. Some combinations have an overall worsening effect on lipids and the lipoprotein profile.

A17 a False
The advantages of inserting the IUCD during menstruation or immediately after a period are that pregnancy is excluded, insertion is easy and any associated bleeding is accepted as normal loss. However, some women prefer not to be examined at this time.

b False
It is important not to remove an IUCD until 1 year after the menopause. At present, it is recommended that inert devices are changed every 4 years and copper devices every 3 years, but this period is likely to be lengthened in the future. The progestin-releasing devices are no longer available, due to the high incidence of ectopic pregnancy.

c True
Provided intercourse has occurred no longer than 5 days previously, an IUCD will prevent implantation. Women should be reviewed after 1 month to check menstruation has occurred and to consider removal of the device.

d True
Spontaneous abortion will occur in about 55% of cases (a 3 times greater incidence than in women without an IUCD). Removal of the IUCD may itself cause abortion, but if this does not happen it will reduce the risk of subsequent abortion. There is no evidence that copper-containing devices cause an increased incidence of fetal abnormality. The device is always extra-amniotic.

e True
Insertion of an IUCD is not a sterile procedure, and the endometrium is colonised following insertion. The risk is higher in nulliparous women. Organisms implicated include chlamydia, gonococcus, anaerobes and, rarely, infection with *Actinomyces israeli*.

A18 a True
Mean menstrual loss is 35 ml, with 95% of women losing less than 60 ml each menses. Menorrhagia is defined as a mean menstrual loss greater than 80 ml, or prolonged (greater than 7 days) menstrual loss. The passage of large clots and flooding indicates a large menstrual loss; however, the woman's own assessment of duration and number of sanitary pads or tampons used correlates poorly with actual blood loss. In about 50% of women with menorrhagia, no cause is found and it is referred to as dysfunctional uterine bleeding. Organic causes include congenital double uterus, IUCD, chronic pelvic inflammatory disease, uterine fibroids, uterine neoplasms and oestrogen-producing ovarian neoplasms. It is also seen with obesity, endometriosis and bleeding disorders.

b True
Non-steroidal anti-inflammatory drugs are prostaglandin synthetase inhibitors. They can reduce menstrual loss by up to 30%. Unfortunately, the benefit decreases over several cycles. Other treatments include: antifibrinolytic agents, danazol, the combined oral contraceptive pill, hysteroscopic transcervical resection of the endometrium and hysterectomy.

c False
Although the incidence of haemorrhage is increased in teenage girls and peri-menopausal women, over 50% are in the 20–40 year age group.

d False

D&C is unlikely to be useful in the treatment of most cases of menorrhagia. It helps only in chronic anovulation (as it removes much of the hyperplastic endometrium) and for endometrial polyps and pedunculated leiomyomas of the uterus (fibroids). It is also useful diagnostically in women over 40 years of age to exclude endometrial carcinoma.

e True

Medical treatment may be used in the interim. The reason for referral is to exclude a pathological cause. The GP should consider performing a full blood count (to exclude anaemia and thrombocytopenia) and a thyroid function test (to exclude hypothyroidism). Sudden changes in menstrual loss should be urgently investigated at this age.

A19 a True

Although figures vary, female causes do seem to predominate. Male factors are being increasingly identified but are more difficult to treat. In many cases, there is a combined cause.

b True

This is a useful test but the result comes several weeks after the event. Luteinising hormone assays are available and will predict ovulation within 12 hours. They are expensive and not routinely available, but commercial kits are available over the counter (e.g. Predictor).

c True

The normal time to conceive increases with age, although it is reasonable to start investigations earlier in older couples.

d True

A history of sub-fertility increases the risk of ectopic pregnancy. This is probably because it identifies a group of women with tubal problems.

e True

Salazopyrin therapy for ulcerative colitis leads to oligospermia. It is reversible on stopping therapy.

A20 a True

Endometriosis is associated with infertility (30–45% of infertile women). Whether this is causal or casual is still debated. There is also an association with women who delay their first pregnancy. It is repeatedly stated in the literature that there is an increase in the higher socioeconomic groups, but this is unlikely to be a true association. There is also no evidence that women of Afro-Caribbean descent have a lower incidence of endometriosis. Inheritance is polygenic; 7% of first degree relatives are affected compared to only 1% of unrelated controls.

b True
This is thought to be due to the greater mean menstrual blood loss with an IUCD, increasing from a normal amount of 35 ml up to 60 ml with small copper devices and 80 ml with a Lippes loop. This results in a greater volume of retrograde menstruation, one of the postulated aetiologies of endometriosis.

c True
Approximately 10% of women with endometriosis have involvement of the urinary tract. Other sites affected include the ovaries, pelvis, bowel, lower genital tract, the umbilicus and abdominal scars. The classic symptoms of endometriosis are cyclical pelvic pain and infertility.

d True
The pill needs to be taken continuously to produce amenorrhoea and 'pseudopregnancy'. The dose may have to be increased to up to 4 tablets per day, but this will produce increased side-effects. Other medical treatments include danazol, luteinising hormone releasing hormone (LHRH) agonists and Gestrinone, a new 19-nortestosterone derivative.

e True
HRT should be given to prevent immediate menopausal symptoms due to oestrogen deficiency, to prevent long-term osteoporosis and, possibly, to reduce the increased risk of ischaemic heart disease.

A21 a True
The risk of miscarriage once a live fetus has been seen on ultrasound is approximately 1 in 200.

b True
Abnormal karyotypes are found in approximately 50% of cases, the most common of which is autosomal trisomy (which accounts for 50%).

c False
There is no evidence that progestogens reduce the risk of miscarriage despite their wide use in general practice. The proposed rationale for using them is that the corpus luteum is the principle source of progesterone during early pregnancy and luteal defects may lead to recurrent miscarriage. However, the lesson of diethylstilboestrol administration for recurrent miscarriage should not be forgotten. This treatment was found to be ineffective and caused vaginal adenocarcinoma in the offspring. There is some evidence that hCG may reduce the risk of recurrent miscarriage but it should not be used until further larger follow-up studies have been performed.

d True
In the community, anti-D is difficult to obtain and as a result is often not given. If the rhesus factor of a patient is not known, then anti-D should be given as a matter of course (50 μg within the first 48 hours). Rhesus disease is preventable, and must not be ignored or forgotten.

e True
Following incomplete abortion, ascending infection may occur. The early signs include raised temperature, abdominal pain, continued bleeding and an offensive vaginal discharge. If infection is suspected, the woman should be admitted to hospital, intravenous antibiotics administered and evacuation performed. Criminal abortion may still need to be considered.

A22 a True

b True
The incidence of osteoporotic fractures may even increase before the menopause. It increases further with increasing age.

c False
They rise to approach male levels, and this helps to explain the increased incidence of cardiovascular disease after the menopause.

d False
It is well absorbed by the vagina and hence will have a systemic effect.

e False
Not in the absence of other risk factors. Whether it should be given to women with a history of thromboembolism is debatable, but in the absence of abnormal clotting the risk appears small.

A23 a True
There is usually abdominal distension from the tumour mass or from accompanying ascites. Ovarian tumours are characteristically symptomless in the early stages. Other recognised symptoms include: dysmenorrhoea, dyspareunia, increase in abdominal girth, increasing weight, acute abdominal pain, lower limb swelling, cachexia and dyspnoea.

b False
The mortality in social class I is twice that in social class V. There is also an association with nulliparity, breast cancer, exposure to talc and asbestos and previous pelvic irradiation. Previous mumps and the combined oral contraceptive pill are believed to have a protective effect.

c False
The majority of patients present as either stage III (growth involving one or both ovaries with intra-peritoneal metastases) or stage IV (growth involving one or both ovaries with distant metastases).

d True
Ovarian cancer accounts for 50% of all deaths from cancer of the female genital tract, but only 25% of gynaecological cancer. In spite of better cytotoxic treatment, the overall five-year survival rate has changed little in recent years and remains at around 25–30%.

e False
The longer the pill is used, the less the likelihood of ovarian cancer. High parity, pregnancy (whether ending in abortion or at term), and breastfeeding all appear to be protective. An early menarche and a late menopause are associated with an increased risk. It appears that ovarian cancer is commoner in women who ovulate for longer.

A24 a True
There is a direct positive correlation between the incidence of secondary amenorrhoea in runners and the number of miles run per week. As training becomes more strenuous, levels of LH and FSH fall significantly.

b False
The majority of women resume ovulatory cycles within 4–6 weeks; however, it is not unusual for a woman to have 1 or 2 months of amenorrhoea before her first menstrual period. Investigation should be considered for more protracted amenorrhoea.

c True
Amenorrhoea traumatica (Asherman's syndrome) may follow D&C, particularly if it has been performed in the puerperium. It is treated by breaking the adhesions via a hysteroscope and inserting an IUCD to keep the uterine walls apart.

d True
Amenorrhoeic women have low levels of oestrogens and this will lead to osteoporosis even before the menopause. Treatment with the contraceptive pill should be considered.

e False
FSH and LH will be raised as there will be no negative feedback on the hypothalamic-pituitary axis. The gonadotrophins are also increased in resistant ovary syndrome. Other investigations should include TSH, prolactin and visual field testing.

A25 a True
Pre-term delivery is defined as delivery before 37 weeks of gestation. Other risk factors include: parity of one or more than four, social class, previous pre-term delivery, ante-partum haemorrhage, multiple pregnancy and, possibly, genital tract infection. Asymptomatic bacteriuria in the absence of renal involvement does not appear to increase the risk of a pre-term delivery. Prevention has thus been largely unsuccessful and the incidence has not changed in recent years.

b False
There is no increased risk providing there is atraumatic cervical dilatation. However, second trimester abortions and stillbirths are risk factors.

c False
Almost any severe maternal illness may be associated with pre-term delivery. Diabetes mellitus is associated with polyhydramnios, congenital abnormalities, hypertension and renal disease.

d False
Although effective treatment for cervical incompetence, cerclage has not been shown to be an effective method of preventing pre-term labour in women at risk.

e True
Most cases of painful contractions settle spontaneously, and tocolytic therapy is unnecessary. The problem is trying to identify the minority who will go on to deliver. If rupture of the membranes has occurred, then pre-term delivery will occur in the vast majority.

A26 a False
Not in themselves, although if they allow the use of steroids or transfer to a neonatal intensive care unit then they will be of help.

b True
They affect the fetal cardiovascular system and can lead to neonatal hyperglycaemia.

c True
Maternal deaths have occurred, particularly if the drugs are given in large volumes of intravenous fluids.

d False
They are the drugs of choice. Beta blockers are potentially dangerous in asthmatics.

e True
Blood sugar must be monitored, and the drugs are relatively contraindicated in diabetics. If they are used, alteration of insulin dosage will be required.

A27 a False
It is only mid-trimester termination that may lead to subsequent miscarriage. Serial examinations are not helpful and a decision regarding a cervical suture should be taken at booking.

b True
Essential for mother, baby and attendants.

c True
Thalassaemia is common, and prenatal diagnosis is offered if both partners have thalassaemia trait. Women with this condition will have a low haemoglobin and should not be given parenteral iron.

d False
The initial promise from uncontrolled studies has not been confirmed by controlled studies. Problems include: extra workload from performing the CTGs, the anxiety induced in the mothers and difficulty in interpretation of antenatal CTGs.

e True
Although not necessary for healthy mothers with singleton pregnancies, iron and folate supplements are recommended for twin pregnancies.

A28 a True
The main problems of HIV infection in pregnancy are that pregnancy may aggravate the course of the disease, and that the disease is transmissible from the mother to the fetus.

b True
Transplacental transmission occurs early in pregnancy. The reported fetal abnormalities include: growth failure, 'box' forehead, wide-set eyes, short nose and patulous lips.

c True
The exact risk is not known, but HIV-positive mothers should be advised to bottle-feed.

d True
Cryptococcus neoformans is the commonest cause of meningitis, bacterial causes being uncommon. If the treatment required is teratogenic, termination should be considered. Other overwhelming opportunistic infections found include *Toxoplasma gondii*, *Cryptosporidium*, *Strongyloides*, *Pneumocystis carinii*, *Herpes simplex*, *Salmonella*, *Aspergillus* and *Mycobacterium avium* and *intracellulare*.

e True
Other tumours associated with HIV infection are Kaposi's sarcoma and Hodgkin's and non-Hodgkin's lymphoma.

A29 a True
Club foot is one of the commonest congenital malformations, occurring in 1 per 1000 live births. Male infants are twice as commonly affected as females (M:F = 2:1). Orthopaedic opinion should be sought, and application of plaster boots recommended, at an early stage. Despite these measures, surgery is necessary in 30% of affected infants before the age of 11.

b False
90% of affected infants are female (M:F = 1:9). Other risk factors include: a positive family history (in 20%), breech delivery (incidence 10 times higher) and first born babies. The incidence is approximately 15 per 10 000 live births. The left hip is affected twice as often as the right. Splinting should commence at 36 hours after birth and be continued for at least 2 months. The orthopaedic surgeon will be involved from an early stage.

c True
Over 80% of affected infants are male (M:F = 5:1). The incidence is 2 per 1000 live births. The risk increases if there is a family history. It should be considered in any infant under 3 months of age presenting with recurrent vomiting. It is suspected clinically by the presence of a palpable abdominal mass during or after a test feed, and the diagnosis may be confirmed by ultrasound or by a barium meal. Treatment is by surgery.

d False
Isolated cleft palate is commoner in females, but cleft palate associated with cleft lip is commoner in males. In 30% of affected infants there is a positive family history. Other risk factors include certain drugs used in pregnancy, such as warfarin and steroids. Considerable parental support is needed, both with counselling and practical aspects of feeding. The lip is normally repaired from the 1st to the 12th week of life, with later repair of the palate at 9 months. Early involvement of a speech therapist is useful.

e True
80% of affected infants are male (M:F = 4:1). The incidence is 1 in 5000 live births, but the condition may take several months to present. The infant is constipated as a result of an aganglionic segment of rectum or colon. Diagnosis can be made by barium enema and confirmed by absence of ganglion cells in a rectal biopsy. Surgical treatment involves resection of the aganglionic segment of large bowel.

A30 a False
Jaundice appearing in the first 24 hours of life is never physiological. The commonest cause will be haemolytic disease. Other causes include congenital infection, maternal drug use, metabolic disorders and biliary atresia.

b False
This level of bilirubin is rarely reached in healthy, term babies. The liver of pre-term infants is less mature and the serum bilirubin will rise much quicker. Treatment will be required sooner.

c False
A positive Coomb's test will lead to haemolysis and then jaundice.

d False
Although extra fluids may be required to avoid dehydration there is no need to insist on full bottle-feeding.

e True
Jaundice affects virtually all pre-term babies to some degree. This is because of the relatively immature liver.

A31 a False
Cyclical ovarian hormonal effects still persist with intact ovaries. However, the exact aetiological cause of pre-menstrual syndrome is not clear.

b True
Support from the medical profession is very important if the woman is to be helped. Medical treatment is unlikely to work without a sympathetic doctor who acknowledges the woman's problems. Counselling and self-help groups are useful.

c True
Aldosterone antagonists are helpful in women whose principle symptoms relate to fluid retention. They do not have any beneficial effect on mood. Spironolactone is usually given in a dose of 25 mg per day from day 18 to day 26 of the cycle. Other treatments include pyridoxine (for mood changes), natural progesterone (for emotional distress and physical symptoms), bromocriptine (for breast tenderness), danazol and diet. LHRH-agonists have been used in refractory cases, but they can only be used for short periods because of the anti-oestrogen effect.

d False
It is defined as cyclical and as having a consistent and predictable relationship to the menses.

e True
The oral contraceptive pill can aggravate symptoms in some women, whilst curing others. It is probably the continuous progestogen use that aggravates PMS and it should therefore be used with caution.

A32 a True
Women initially have irregular uterine bleeding but most develop complete amenorrhoea. One-third are amenorrhoeic within one year. Depoprovera is not licensed for use in the USA, partly because an increased incidence of breast cancer has been found in beagles. This association has not been found in humans. In the USA Depoprovera is used in the treatment of endometriosis and endometrial cancer.

b False
It is recommended for use in women with sickle cell anaemia. The disease actually improves, with fewer sickle crises and a rise in serum haemoglobin. Oestrogens are contraindicated in sickle cell anaemia.

c True
Medroxyprogesterone (150 mg i.m., 3-monthly) is probably even more effective than the combined oral contraceptive pill. Care must be taken to ensure that the woman is not pregnant before starting the treatment. Its main disadvantages are irregular menstruation initially, weight gain and some delay (up to 18 months) in the restoration of ovulation when the treatment is discontinued.

d True
Minute amounts are excreted in breast milk, but no adverse effects have been found. In fact, there is evidence to suggest that the quality and quantity of milk produced is increased.

e True
It is important to warn patients of this possible problem.

A33 a True
Chorionic villus biopsy is becoming more widely available for pre-natal diagnosis. Although its main advantage is that it can be used in the first trimester, it can still be used after 12 weeks. A technician is available to confirm that enough tissue has been obtained.

b True
Cystic fibrosis can be diagnosed on chorionic villi by restriction fragment length polymorphism. This requires genetic material from the two carriers (i.e. parents) and from the previously affected child.

c True
DNA analysis of villi can diagnose male fetuses affected by haemophilia.

d True
Chromosome analysis of the villi can usually be done within 24 hours, as the cells do not need to be cultured. Since this condition is commoner in women over 35, it may be diagnosed if CVS is done for this reason.

e True
Fragile X is the most common cause of mental retardation in males after Down's syndrome. When fragile X mental retardation has been established within a family, prenatal testing should be carried out on at-risk fetuses.

A34 a False
4%, i.e. 1 in 25. The background incidence of spina bifida is 2 per 1000 births. Other causes of raised maternal serum alpha-fetoprotein include: anencephaly, fetal anterior wall defects, congenital nephrosis, posterior urethral valves, Turner's syndrome, trisomy 13, oesophageal atresia, duodenal atresia, miscarriage and intra-uterine death.

b True
Women with insulin-dependent diabetes tend to have low maternal serum AFP and a high risk of pregnancy affected by a neural tube defect. A cut-off lower than that in the general population is used in this group of women.

c False
Fetuses with Down's syndrome produce less AFP than normal. This can be used to estimate the risk of Down's, which increases with advancing maternal age. It is 1 in 350 at 35 years, 1 in 100 at 40 years and 1 in 30 at 45 years.

d True
This is performed to confirm gestational age and to look for the causes of a raised serum AFP. Often, a repeat AFP is performed before amniocentesis. The risks to the fetus must be considered before amniocentesis is carried out. In experienced hands, there is an estimated excess risk of 0.8% of fetal loss due to this procedure.

e True
Intra-uterine death is associated with very high serum AFP levels. Vaginal bleeding early in pregnancy is also associated with high serum AFP, even if the pregnancy does not end in miscarriage.

A35 a True
Approximately 2–3% of babies present by the breech at term. This incidence is not altered by external cephalic version unless it is performed after 38 weeks.

b True
This is important if considering elective caesarean section, and an ultrasound should be performed for fetal anomaly if not previously done.

c True
The rate of cord prolapse with breech presentations is about 4%. This is mainly due to the increased incidence with flexed and footling breeches. The rate for extended breech presentation is similar to vertex presentations (0.3%).

d False
There is no link with postpartum haemorrhage per se. Obviously, the blood loss will be greater if caesarean section is required.

e True
Although there used to be a significificant perinatal mortality from trauma in breech deliveries, this was mainly due to the practice of breech extraction. This has been abandoned (except for the second twin) and hence traumatic deaths are rare.

A36 a False
The employer must be informed at least 21 days before the woman intends to leave work. The woman should supply the employer with the medical evidence of when the baby is due. This is in the form of a certificate (MAT B1), which is supplied by either the GP or the midwife. Full information is given in leaflet FB8, 'Babies and Benefits' obtainable from a social security office.

b False
The form MAT B1(A) is issued by the GP or midwife not earlier than 14 weeks before the expected week of delivery (i.e. after 26 weeks of pregnancy).

c True
This will depend on her National Insurance contributions. The woman should inform the DSS and supply them with the completed MAT B1 and MA1 forms. If she is employed, she should also submit a form SMP 1 from her employer stating why the employer will not pay SMP. Maternity allowance (as with SMP) is paid for 18 weeks starting from the 11th week before the baby is due.

d True
MAT B1(A) is used before confinement and form MAT B1(B) after confinement. If the woman cannot get either SMP from her employer or maternity allowance from social services she is still able to receive sickness benefit. The form MAT B1(A) is accepted as evidence of incapacity for work for the period starting 6 weeks before the birth of the baby, and ending 2 weeks after the actual date of the birth.

e True
NHS prescriptions are also free.

A37 a False
Chlamydia trachomatis now appears to have taken over in the UK and in Scandinavia. Both organisms are often present together, and the rule that when one sexually transmitted disease is found others should be looked for applies. *Gonococcus* and *Chlamydia* are also the causes of the uncommon 'Fitz-Hugh-Curtis syndrome' of peri-hepatitis. In this syndrome, there is an exudative inflammation of the liver capsule secondary to pelvic infection. It can mimic acute cholecystitis.

b True
The main differential diagnosis of bilateral pelvic tenderness is endometriosis, which can only be excluded by laparoscopy. Laparoscopy also allows checking of tubal patency.

c True
Other sequelae of PID include chronic pelvic pain, dyspareunia, menorrhagia, dysmenorrhoea and ectopic pregnancy (an increased risk of up to 10-fold).

d True
The placental site is an ideal culture medium for infecting organisms. The usual organisms in this situation are *E.coli*, *Clostridia*, *Streptococci* and *Staphylococci*.

e True
No single drug covers all the organisms involved. The choice of antibiotic regime depends on the likely cause. Culture for *Chlamydia* may take several days and is best presumed to be present unless proven otherwise. Tetracycline is the treatment of choice and should be continued for at least 14 days.

A38 a False
Mild ketoacidosis is often found in diabetic pregnant women treated by diet alone and is not regarded as harmful. Gestational diabetes is usually treated with diet alone. Regular blood sugars should be monitored by the woman and the antenatal clinic. If diet fails to control blood sugars insulin therapy should be added. Oral hypoglycaemic agents cross the placenta and induce fetal hyperinsulinaemia.

b False

Glycosuria is very common in pregnancy due to less efficient renal tubular re-absorption. Blood sugar estimations are required to accurately screen for diabetes; they can be performed at random times and the results interpreted with reference to the last meal (e.g. 6.4 mmol/l less than 2 hours after a meal or 5.8 mmol/l at any other time).

c False

Fructosamine and glycosylated haemoglobin (Hb A_1) are used to monitor control in insulin dependent diabetics but are not suitable as a screening test. They indicate past levels of serum glucose rather than present levels.

d False

Although 100 g tests are used in the USA, British, European and WHO criteria for the diagnosis of diabetes require a 75 g oral glucose tolerance test.

e True

Other risk factors for gestational diabetes include fasting glycosuria, polyhydramnios and a previous history of gestational diabetes, macrosomia or unexplained stillbirth.

A39 a False

Babies who are allowed to feed on demand put on more weight and continue breastfeeding longer. Interestingly, there is no increased incidence of cracked nipples with longer duration of feeds.

b False

Breastfeeding should be continued, with particular attention given to correct positioning of the baby. Mastitis is best treated with flucloxacillin (500 mg orally q.d.s. for 5 days). The condition results from excess collections of milk in the breast alveoli, and can progress to infection and abcess formation. When this occurs, the woman develops systemic symptoms with shivering attacks, rigors, headaches and flu-like symptoms.

c False

There is no evidence that increased fluid intake improves lactation. In fact, the increased urine output may cause distress to women with perineal and labial trauma.

d False

There is no evidence that starting breastfeeding later (4 hours after the birth) is better or worse than starting early (immediately after delivery). It is more important that the women receive appropriate and practical help and support.

e True

Although the evidence is not totally consistent, the duration of breastfeeding has been shown to be increased in women who have regular and frequent contacts with appropriate carers.

A40 a True
It is likely to be physiological. The mean duration of lochia is 33 days, with 13% of women still having persistent lochia at 60 days. If bleeding continues to decrease progressively, it is likely to be normal.

b True
The progestogen-only pill (POP) causes more breakthrough bleeding the earlier in the puerperium it is used, and for this reason may be discontinued by the woman. 50% fewer women discontinue treatment because of bleeding problems if the POP is commenced at 6 weeks post-partum compared with women who started it at 1 week post-partum. However, to reduce the risk of early fertile ovulation it is probably best started in the 3rd to 4th week of the puerperium.

c False
If the bleeding is significant and increasing, a gynaecological opinion should be sought. Endometrial pathology is rare at 4 weeks, since retained products and infection will usually have presented by then. Curettage may occasionally be required, but must be performed by an experienced operator since perforation is more common than in the non-pregnant.

d True
This is excessively rare 4 weeks post delivery.

e True
The incidence is difficult to assess; however, the cervix must always be visualised.

3. Paper B

B1 Which of the following are features of the polycystic ovary syndrome?:
a Multiple pregnancies
b Hair loss
c Virilisation
d Anorexia nervosa
e Menorrhagia

B2 Regarding termination of pregnancy in the UK:
a The majority are done under Section 1 of the 1967 Abortion Act
b Vacuum aspiration is safer the later the gestation
c A GP who has a conscientious objection may opt out of referring a woman for an abortion
d It is illegal to refer and perform an abortion on a minor without parental consent
e Women presenting for termination have often had a previous termination

B3 The following conditions suggest that booking in a GP unit would be unwise:
a Previous hysterotomy
b Previous postpartum haemorrhage
c Previous lift-out forceps delivery
d A previous D&C
e An 18-year old primigravida

B4 Placental abruption:
a Is a less common cause of third trimester bleeding than placenta praevia
b Is always due to rupture of spiral arteries beneath the placenta
c Is predisposed to by cocaine abuse in pregnancy
d The risk of recurrence is greater in smokers
e May be recognised on ultrasound

B5   Trichomonas vaginalis vaginal infection:
a Is usually sexually transmitted
b Often occurs with gonorrhoea
c Is treated with penicillin
d Can be diagnosed by a characteristic ammonia smell when the discharge is mixed with 10% potassium chloride
e Does not require treatment

B6   Antepartum haemorrhage (APH):
a Is defined as bleeding from the genital tract after 20 weeks' gestation
b Can be caused by cervical polyps
c Can be managed at home if the bleeding is slight
d Increases the risk of a postpartum haemorrhage (PPH)
e Should have a vaginal digital examination performed immediately

B7   Asymptomatic bacteriuria during pregnancy:
a Does not usually require any treatment
b Requires investigation by IVU after delivery
c Occurs in 5% of pregnant women
d Is usually caused by beta haemolytic streptococci
e May lead to pyelonephritis

B8   In the management of a prolapsed umbilical cord occurring at home which of the following statements are true?:
a No intervention should be attempted until the arrival of the flying squad
b The condition is more common with twins
c The cord should be placed gently back into the vagina
d Catheterisation to empty the woman's bladder should be performed
e The woman should be stood upright to aid immediate delivery

B9   Prostaglandin PGE_2 intravaginal pessaries used in the induction of labour:
a Should be placed in the cervical canal
b Do not promote cervical ripening in women with low Bishop scores
c May induce fetal distress
d Should be continued indefinitely until artificial rupture of the membranes (ARM) can be performed
e May produce uterine hypertonia

B10 Premature rupture of membranes:
   a Is defined as the leakage of amniotic fluid prior to the onset of contractions at any stage of pregnancy up to 40 weeks
   b Amniotic fluid is detected by turning nitrazine yellow
   c Digital vaginal examination must be performed
   d Prophylactic antibiotics decrease neonatal infections
   e Corticosteroids are contraindicated because of the risk of infection

B11 Constipation in pregnancy:
   a Is a result of delayed gastrointestinal motility
   b Liquid paraffin is contraindicated
   c Should not be treated with Senna
   d May cause acute abdominal pain
   e Is exacerbated by iron therapy

B12 Concerning puberty in girls:
   a The hypothalamus plays a major role in the onset of puberty
   b The appearance of pubic hair is the first sign
   c The average age of the menarche has fallen
   d Breast development usually starts by 11 years of age
   e Most cases of precocious puberty are pathological

B13 Which of the following conditions are contraindications to the combined oral contraceptive pill?:
   a Varicose veins
   b Otosclerosis
   c Family history of diabetes mellitus
   d Breastfeeding
   e Depression

B14 Laparoscopic sterilisation:
   a In the UK, requires consent from both the husband and wife
   b Is unlikely to be successfully reversed when Filshie clips have been used
   c A period of 3 months after the operation is necessary before it can be presumed all ova have been eliminated from the fallopian tubes
   d Causes menorrhagia
   e Has a higher failure rate if the procedure is performed immediately postpartum

B15 Which of the following clinical symptoms occur with an ectopic pregnancy?:
   a Vaginal bleeding
   b Amenorrhoea
   c Shoulder tip pain
   d Dizziness
   e Recurrent abdominal pain

B16 A sperm sample is abnormal if:
   a The volume is 1 ml³
   b The sperm concentration is 5 million/ml³
   c 45% of sperm have forward motility
   d 50% of sperm have normal oval forms
   e There are more than 10 white blood cells (wbc) per high powered field

B17 Instrumental delivery in a GP unit should not be attempted if:
   a The cervix is 9 cm dilated
   b The head is not palpable abdominally
   c The membranes are intact
   d The woman has not been catheterised
   e The position of the presenting part has not been determined

B18 The second stage of labour:
   a Normally lasts no longer than 1 hour in primigravida, and 30 minutes in multigravida
   b Causes flexion and internal rotation of the head at delivery
   c Should be conducted in the lithotomy position in primigravida
   d Is more likely to end with forceps with an epidural in situ
   e May be heralded by vomiting

B19 Stress incontinence:
   a Is more common in nulliparous women
   b Is best treated by terodolin
   c May be prevented by para-urethral pressure during pelvic examination
   d Is unlikely to occur with urge incontinence
   e Has been shown to be prevented by pelvic floor exercises post delivery

B20 Vulval warts:
   a Are usually spread by sexual contact
   b Are unaffected by pregnancy
   c Are best treated with podophyllin during pregnancy
   d Are implicated in cancer of the cervix
   e Can be transmitted to a neonate during birth

B21 An elderly woman with pruritus vulvae presenting to her GP:
   a Requires a full blood count
   b Should have a urine test for glucose
   c Should be referred for vulval biopsy if leukoplakia is present
   d May have psoriasis
   e Should have a high vaginal swab taken

B22 Anovulation as a cause of subfertility may be treated in general practice by:
   a Weight gain in women with a low body mass index
   b Danazol
   c Clomiphene
   d Pergonal
   e Bromocriptine

B23 A 19-year-old girl who has never had a period:
   a Requires a vaginal examination
   b May be normal
   c Requires FSH/LH estimation
   d Should have a skull X-ray on presentation
   e Should have chromosomal evaluation

B24 Rhesus iso-immunisation:
   a No longer occurs due to the use of Anti-D
   b Would be prevented by measuring maternal antibodies
   c May occur antenatally in primigravida
   d May require intra-uterine blood transfusion for the fetus
   e Gets better with each pregnancy

B25 Pelvic pain in a woman of 35 years may be due to:
   a Ovulation
   b Irritable bowel syndrome
   c Ectopic pregnancy
   d Endometriosis
   e Appendicitis

B26 Vomiting at 10 weeks of pregnancy may be a symptom of:
   a Hyperemesis gravidarum
   b Pyelonephritis
   c Torsion of an ovarian cyst
   d A degenerating fibroid
   e Severe pre-eclampsia

B27 Uterovaginal prolapse:
   a Is termed procidentia when the cervix lies outside the introitus
   b May be asymptomatic
   c Is best treated by a ring pessary
   d May cause retention of urine
   e Is prevented by liberal use of episiotomy at delivery

B28 As a GP, one of your patients has been treated for a hydatidiform mole. Which of the following advice is correct?:
  a The combined oral contraceptive pill must not be used for 1 year
  b Pregnancy should be avoided for 12 months
  c After treatment the risk of recurrence is the same as for a non-affected woman
  d Congenital abnormalities are commoner in subsequent pregnancies
  e Uterine pain in the first 2 weeks following evacuation is unlikely to be significant

B29 Cytological screening for carcinoma of the cervix:
  a Has not reduced the mortality in the UK
  b Can stop at 70 years of age if regular smears have previously been normal
  c Produces a large number of minor abnormalities in normal women
  d Under the new GP contract, a GP is eligible for the higher payment if 80% of his women patients aged 25–64 years have had a smear within the last 5½ years
  e Is best done on day 21 of the menstrual cycle

B30 Maternal mortality:
  a Only includes deaths from abortion, pregnancy and labour up to 42 days after delivery
  b Occurs at a rate of 1 every 10 000 births in the UK
  c Is most commonly due to hypertensive disease
  d Due to thromboembolism, is commoner in multiparous women over 35 years of age
  e Due to caesarean section, is 5 times greater in emergency than elective section

B31 A retroverted uterus:
  a Is usually a normal finding
  b Is a common cause of dyspareunia
  c Is likely to become incarcerated during pregnancy
  d May be due to endometriosis
  e Can be surgically treated by laparoscopic methods

B32 Karyotype 46XX is compatible with:
  a Turner's syndrome
  b Klinefelter's syndrome
  c Down's syndrome
  d Treacher Collins syndrome
  e Marfan's syndrome

B33 The features of Down's syndrome include:
   a Posterior atlanto-occipital subluxation
   b A double palmar crease
   c Koplik's spots
   d An increased incidence of acute leukaemia
   e An association with tetralogy of Fallot

B34 If a baby delivered at home has a fit, which of the following should be performed at the bedside?:
   a Administration of high concentration oxygen
   b Heel blood estimate of blood glucose
   c Removal of all covers from the neonate
   d Always arrange immediate admission
   e Administration of intramuscular benzylpenicillin

B35 Maternal shock in labour may be due to:
   a Uterine rupture
   b Amniotic fluid embolism
   c Pulmonary embolism
   d Blood transfusion
   e Uterine inversion

B36 At the 6-week post natal examination:
   a The FP24 should be completed
   b Vaginal examination is essential
   c Elevated blood pressure due to pre-eclampsia will usually have returned to normal
   d Coils can be inserted without concern about further pregnancy
   e Smears are only reliable after caesarean section, and not after vaginal delivery

B37 Fetal blood pH estimation in labour:
   a Is more accurate than cardiotocographs in predicting fetal acidosis
   b A pH of 7.25 is normal
   c Must be performed in the lithotomy position
   d Is not affected if liquor is mixed with the blood
   e Can not be obtained in breech presentations

B38 Retained placenta:
   a May be due to placenta accreta
   b Can be left until 24 hours after delivery
   c Will increase post-partum blood loss
   d May require hysterotomy
   e Is more likely after a previous caesarean section

B39 Which of the following are true of epidural anaesthesia in labour?:
   a Increased frequency of instrumental delivery
   b Increased incidence of hypotension
   c It causes urinary incontinence
   d It causes headache
   e It causes incoordinate uterine contraction

B40 Which of the following lead to infants who are small for gestational age?:
   a Diabetes
   b Postmaturity
   c Pre-eclampsia
   d Smoking
   e Working after 28 weeks of pregnancy

4. Paper B Answers

B1 **a False**
Anovulatory infertility occurs in 75% of women with polycystic ovary syndrome. It was first described by Stein and Leventhal in 1935. The aetiology is unclear. Due to the lack of an LH surge spontaneous ovulation does not occur, but can be induced by clomiphene. This may be associated with multiple pregnancy. Biochemical features include elevated serum LH, oestrogen and androgen levels, with a high LH/FSH ratio.

b False
70% of women with polycystic ovary syndrome develop hirsutism (excessive facial and body hair). It is due to excess androgens. Treatment with the combined oral contraceptive pill is effective, but may take several months to work. Cyproterone acetate is an anti-androgen and results in substantial improvement in 70% of women; however, it reduces libido, affects the liver and can interfere with the development of a male fetus (so pregnancy must be avoided). Wedge resection of the ovaries does not help hirsutism.

c True
Virilisation is defined as the presence of one or more of the following; clitoral hypertrophy, breast atrophy, male-type baldness and deepening of the voice. It is a rare manifestation of polycystic ovary syndrome. Treatment is as in **b**, i.e. suppressing the excess androgens. The GP may be of particular help in counselling the woman, especially with these distressing androgenic symptoms.

d False
The initial description of a woman with the polycystic ovary syndrome was of an obese, hirsute, infertile female with oligomenorrhoea and bilaterally enlarged polycystic ovaries. However, it is now clear that obesity is not as common as at first thought. Obese women with the syndrome are helped by weight loss, as this reduces the amount of peripheral conversion of androgens to oestrogens.

e False

Oligomenorrhoea is the clinical feature. These women are also at risk of endometrial carcinoma due to excessive unopposed oestrogen stimulation. The combined oral contraceptive pill is therapeutic and preventative.

B2 a False

Section 1 states that continuation of pregnancy would involve risk to the life of the pregnant woman greater than that if the pregnancy were terminated. Only 0.5% of induced abortions are performed for this reason. The majority (86%) are performed under section 2, which states that continuation of the pregnancy would involve risk of injury to the physical or mental health of the pregnant woman greater than would be involved if the pregnancy were terminated.

b False

Generally, suction curettage is used for first-trimester abortion only. The complications include perforation of the uterus, haemorrhage and infection. Fully documented counselling of the woman prior to termination is important for medico-legal reasons. In the second trimester, prostaglandins are mainly used to induce uterine contractions to expel the fetus.

c True

The GP has a responsibility to assist the woman to obtain alternative medical advice. If the doctor does not conscientiously oppose abortion, he or she must make a clinical decision concerning the risks of abortion against those of continuing the pregnancy. The 1967 Abortion Act requires that two doctors sign the green form (Form HSA 1) and, between them, decide if a woman has grounds for abortion.

d False

It is not illegal to perform an abortion on a girl under 16 years of age without parental consent, but it is inadvisable. Similarly, a termination should not be performed if it is contrary to the girl's wishes, even if her parents demand it. Teenagers, unfortunately, often present later in pregnancy for termination.

e False

Only 9% of abortions are repeat operations. It is a myth that women use it as a means of contraception.

B3 a True

Women who have had hysterotomy are at risk from uterine rupture, and must be managed in hospital under consultant care. Any previous gynaecological operations, e.g. myomectomy or cone biopsy, put the pregnancy at risk.

b True
A PPH in a previous pregnancy increases the risk of a further PPH. Other absolute contraindications to delivery in a GP unit include: caesarean section, previous retained placenta, intra-uterine growth retardation, diabetes or other maternal illness, pelvic injury and multiple pregnancy. Relative contraindications may include infertility treatment and a history of recurrent miscarriages.

c False
A difficult delivery involving mid-cavity forceps is a relative contraindication to delivery in a GP unit. Other relative contraindications include: primigravida, small multigravida (less than 150 cm tall), fifth or more baby, and multigravida over 40.

d False
It is important to ask if uterine perforation occurred, as this may increase the risk of uterine rupture in pregnancy.

e True
Young (less than 18-year-old) primigravida should be considered for consultant unit booking. They are at increased risk of low birthweight babies and have a high rate of transfer in labour for conditions such as dysfunctional labour and for epidural analgesia.

B4 a False
Placenta praevia accounts for 10%, and abruptions 15–20% of antepartum haemorrhages.

b False
Retroplacental haemorrhage results from rupture of spiral arteries, and marginal haemorrhage from tears of the marginal veins.

c True
Other risk factors include smoking, raised serum alpha fetoprotein and increasing age and parity. The relationship with hypertension remains unclear.

d True
Hence, the woman should be strongly urged to stop smoking.

e True
Although this is not a reliable method of definitive diagnosis, a localised haematoma may be recognised by ultrasound.

B5 a True
Trichomonas vaginalis is usually, but not always, transmitted by sexual contact. Treatment is not complete until the woman's sexual partner has been treated. If he is not treated as well, there is a failure rate of 24%. During treatment, a sheath should be used during intercourse.

b True
When one sexually transmitted disease is found, others frequently coexist and should be looked for. This principle is extremely important.

c False
Oral metronidazole is the treatment of choice, either 200 mg orally tds for 7 days, 800 mg orally bd for 1 day or 2 g as a single dose. Alcohol should be avoided with metronidazole. During pregnancy, metronidazole is not advised during the first 3 months, even though there is no evidence of teratogenicity. During this time, local agents and sheaths during intercourse are used instead, together with local hygiene.

d False
This fishy smell is produced by the *Gardnerella vaginalis*.

e False
It is sexually transmitted and will give rise to symptoms if not treated. It does not, however, lead to systemic disease.

B6 a False
APH is traditionally defined as any bleeding from the genital tract from 28 completed weeks of pregnancy until the birth of the baby. It therefore includes the first and second stages of labour. In recent years, it has become clear that babies of even 24 weeks are capable of survival. Furthermore, the causes can clearly manifest before 28 weeks and, in practice, bleeding after 22 weeks is managed as an obstetric problem rather than as a threatened miscarriage. It complicates 3% of pregnancies progressing beyond 28 weeks gestation.

b True
The causes of APH are classified as placental abruption, placenta praevia, lesions of the cervix and vagina, and indeterminate. The group of indeterminate causes includes marginal haemorrhage from the placenta which has no positive clinical features. Placental abruption causes painful bleeding, while the other causes are usually painless.

c False
All women should be admitted to hospital and investigated. Maternal blood is taken for haemoglobin estimation, platelet count, the Kleihauer test (which demonstrates fetal erythrocytes in maternal blood) and crossmatching. If abruption is suspected, clotting studies should also be performed to exclude disseminated intravascular coagulation (DIC). An ultrasound scan should be performed to exclude placenta praevia. If excluded, a speculum examination is then performed to exclude lower genital tract bleeding. If the bleeding is slight and settles, the woman will be allowed home. Anti-D should be given to rhesus-negative women.

d True
The incidence of PPH is increased after an APH.

e False
The cardinal rule is NEVER perform a vaginal examination on a woman with an undiagnosed APH, as placenta praevia may be present.

B7 a False
Asymptomatic bacteriuria is significant if there are 10^5 organisms per ml of cultured urine. If untreated, these women are 4 times more likely to develop symptomatic urinary infection than are women without bacteriuria. It is no longer thought that asymptomatic bacteriuria is associated with low birthweight, fetal loss, pre-eclampsia and maternal anaemia. It must be treated with an agent effective against the responsible organism, but also one that is safe for use in pregnancy, e.g. ampicillin or a cephalosporin.

b False
Although 2% of pregnant women with asymptomatic bacteriuria will have some abnormality of the urinary tract, it is usually minor. Intravenous urography should be considered following delivery in those women who develop acute recurrent symptomatic infections, in those in whom the bacteriuria persists despite treatment and in those who develop recurrence postpartum.

c True
2% of non-pregnant and 5–7% of pregnant women have asymptomatic bacteriuria.

d False
Over 90% are caused by *E.coli*. Other organisms responsible include *Klebsiella*, *Proteus*, *Staphylococci* and *Psuedomonas*.

e True
15–45% of untreated asymptomatic women will develop a symptomatic infection during pregnancy. Pyelonephritis must be treated in hospital with intravenous antibiotics. Ampicillin or cephalosporins are appropriate treatments unless the woman is seriously ill, when gentamicin should be combined with ampicillin.

B8 a False
The presenting part should be pushed back into the uterus, and the woman instructed to adopt a knee-elbow position. If a catheter is available, the bladder should be filled with 750 ml of normal saline. The obstetric flying squad should be called immediately. Immediate forceps delivery should only be attempted if the GP is sufficiently experienced, and the cervix is fully dilated.

b True
Consequently, and because of the increased risks of prematurity, women living large distances from obstetric units should be admitted in late pregnancy. No woman with multiple pregnancy should be booked for home delivery. Cord prolapse is associated with a high presenting part at the time of rupture of the membranes.

c True
This is done because the vagina is at a higher temperature than the surrounding air and will prevent vasospasm of the cord. However, great care must be taken not to cause vasospasm by manipulation.

d False
See **a**. If the bladder is empty, the presenting part is likely to descend further into the pelvis and compress the cord.

e False
As with **d**, the presenting part will compress the cord and cause fetal asphyxia. If the woman is fully dilated, however, delivery may be possible by adequate maternal effort.

B9 a False
Prostaglandin pessaries are placed in the posterior fornix. Preparations are available for intra-cervical use, but they are not widely used in the UK.

b False
This is their main use in modern obstetrics. Induction is sometimes required in the face of an unfavourable cervix, and prostaglandins can help avoid caesarean section. They can also be used to induce labour in the presence of a favourable cervix.

c True
This is a potential response of the fetus to contractions and therefore monitoring should be used once contractions start.

d False
If delivery is required, then some time limit has to be set, and so either an amniotomy or a caesarean section will have to be performed.

e True
This may compromise the fetus and adversely affect the outcome. Monitoring of the mother and fetus is important.

B10 a False
Premature rupture of the membranes is defined as occurring after 20 and before 37 completed weeks of gestation. In 8% of all pregnancies, the membranes rupture prematurely. The main problems encountered are cord prolapse, ascending infection and premature labour.

b False
Amniotic fluid leakage has a slightly alkaline pH of 7–7.5, which causes nitrazine to change from yellow to blue. However blood, urine, lubricants or antiseptic solutions may produce false-positive results.

c False
Digital examination is to be avoided unless it has been decided to proceed with labour. Sterile speculum examination is used to estimate cervical dilatation and degree of effacement, as well as to obtain fluid for confirmation of rupture and microscopy. Gross cord prolapse is also excluded.

d False
In controlled trials, there has been no reduction in the incidence of neonatal infection or maternal infection before delivery. The only significant finding is that maternal postpartum infections are reduced in incidence. This may equally apply if the antibiotics are started at delivery instead of before.

e False
Although there is a slight increase in the incidence of neonatal infection, the effect is smaller than the lower incidence of respiratory distress syndrome produced by corticosteroid administration.

B11 a True
Bowel transit time increases in the first and second trimesters, but returns to non-pregnant levels in the third trimester. It affects up to 30% of women. Important factors include: the effect of progesterone on the bowel, reduced fibre intake due to pica (cravings), iron treatment and further exacerbation by increased water absorption from the gut due to the prolonged transit time.

b True
Malabsorption of fat soluble vitamins may occur.

c True
Stimulant laxatives may produce uterine contractions in sensitive individuals. Increasing dietary fibre, regular exercise and bulking agents are all useful remedies.

d True
Other common causes of abdominal pain in pregnancy include: placental abruption, abortion, ectopic pregnancy, fibroid degeneration, uterine rupture, ovarian cyst torsion, appendicitis, renal colic and pyelonephritis.

e True
Oral iron supplements, e.g. ferrous sulphate, Pregaday, all cause or worsen constipation. Appropriate dietary advice should be given.

B12 a True
Maturation of the hypothalamic neuroendocrine mechanism is responsible for the control of pituitary gonadotrophin secretion and, hence, that of the ovary. There is some evidence that the pineal gland also has an important role.

b False
The development of the breast bud occurs first at approximately 11 years of age. Initially this may be asymmetrical but only lasts for a short time.

c True
The mean age of the menarche is now 12.5 years, with a range of 10 to 16 years.

d True

e False
The development of secondary sex characteristics before the age of 8 is precocious. In boys, 50% have a space-occupying lesion of the CNS, but in girls 75–90% are idiopathic.

B13 a False
Varicose veins are a relative contraindication to the oral contraceptive pill as they are worsened. Other relative contraindications include known risk factors for arterial disease, smoking, age, immobilization, hyperprolactinaemia and oligomenorrhoea.

b True
Otosclerosis is known to be worsened by the pill or pregnancy. Other absolute contraindications are arterial or venous thrombosis, transient ischaemic attacks, focal migraine, liver disease, oestrogen-dependent cancer, pregnancy, undiagnosed genital tract bleeding, recent trophoblastic disease and major surgery.

c False
Diabetes itself is not a contraindication to the use of the combined oral contraceptive pill, provided there are no vascular complications. The pill is thought to accelerate retinopathy and small vessel disease. Although the pill has a slight effect on carbohydrate tolerance, it does not usually increase insulin requirements. The main problem is a slight increase in the risk of thromboembolism. The progestogen-only pill or an intra-uterine contraceptive device may be preferable.

d False *True*
The combined pill reduces the amount of milk produced and is a relative contraindication. Barrier methods or the progestogen-only pill are the methods of choice.

e False
Very severe depression is a relative contraindication to the pill. Depression is more likely with high dose preparations than low dose oestrogen pills.

B14 a False
Whilst with all sterilisation procedures it is preferable to counsel both partners, consent is only required from the woman.

b False
In experienced hands, 75% of clip sterilisations can be successfully reversed. However, the woman should be counselled pre-operatively that the aim of the operation is to be irreversible.

c False

It is advisable that women use contraception at least up to the day of operation. If methods of contraception are used which do not prevent ovulation, contraceptive measures should still be employed until menstruation occurs, as there may be an ovum already in the uterus. Following vasectomy, men may take a considerable time before they become azoospermic, and two negative semen samples should be obtained.

d False

If the woman has been on the combined pill, she should be advised that her periods will increase due to withdrawal of this method as she reverts back to her natural menstruation.

e True

The pregnancy rate post-partum is 1.4 per 100 women per year, compared with a rate for interval sterilisation of 0.4. Immediately post-partum is not the best time to make decisions about potentially irreversible sterilisation.

B15 a True

75% have some degree of abnormal bleeding. An ectopic pregnancy should always be considered when bleeding occurs in early pregnancy, particularly when there is unilateral abdominal pain. Bleeding is usually mild, but can be misleadingly heavy due to loss of decidual cast. Pelvic examination should not be performed at home if an ectopic is the likely diagnosis. An intravenous infusion should be set up, and the woman admitted to hospital.

b True

25% of women with ectopic pregnancy have not experienced any alteration in menstruation.

c True

This is due to free blood irritating the diaphragm. Cullen's sign (periumbilical darkening) may be found.

d True

This is produced by hypovolaemia due to intraperitoneal bleeding, and should not be ignored in a pregnant woman.

e True

Subacute ectopic bleeding can be difficult to diagnose. Dizziness, shoulder tip pain and pain on defaecation (due to blood in the pouch of Douglas) should all be enquired about.

B16 a True

Normal volume is 2–6 ml. Semen should be tested at least 2 days after abstinence. It is best obtained by induced ejaculation, but can be obtained by intercourse using withdrawal. Rubber condoms should not be used as spermatozoa may be killed. The sample should arrive in the laboratory within 1 hour.

b True
Normal fertile is greater than 20 million/ml^3; subfertile is between 5 and 20 million/ml^3; and infertile is less than 5 million/ml^3.

c True
60% or more should have forward motility within 2 hours. Before this abnormality is confirmed, two further samples should be analysed.

d True
60% or more should have normal morphology. As above, 3 samples should be analysed.

e True
More than 5 wbc per high power field suggests prostatitis. This should be treated by a 3-month course of antibiotics, and the count then repeated.

B17 a True
The cervix must be fully dilated, or considerable maternal damage can be done.

b False
Before embarking on forceps, the abdomen should be palpated. Even if there is no head palpable, vaginal delivery may not be possible due to mid-cavity or outlet obstruction. It is probably wisest to confine forceps deliveries in GP units to lift-out forceps, i.e. when the head is on the perineum.

c True
The membranes should be ruptured and then the forceps may be unnecessary.

d False
As the bladder is an intra-abdominal organ, it will not obstruct delivery when the head is through the pelvis (lift-out forceps). For a mid-cavity forceps delivery, the woman is catheterised prior to and after delivery to exclude pre-existing bladder trauma and to check that it has not occurred during the procedure. There may be an increased risk of introducing infection into the bladder.

e True
Only those with a known occipito-anterior position should be attempted.

B18 a True
These are the generally accepted maximum lengths. This does not mean that intervention has to be undertaken at this stage, particularly in primips, providing the fetus is monitored, the mother is keen to carry on and progress is occurring. In multiparous women, failure to deliver after 30 minutes may indicate a malposition, e.g. a brow presentation.

b False
Delivery of the fetal head occurs by extension. Once the head is delivered, restitution follows by external rotation.

c False
This is only necessary when forceps have to be applied. It may also be advisable for breech deliveries.

d True
This can be reduced by allowing longer in the second stage and starting oxytocin if the head does not reach the pelvic floor spontaneously.

e True
This is probably due to vagal stimulation. The bradycardia quickly resolves, and normal pushing can be allowed. It tends not to occur with an epidural.

B19 a False
Stress incontinence is more common in multiparous women and during pregnancy, but it does occur in nulliparous women. Both fast and long labours, as well as large babies, are thought to be causative factors. The prevalence among nulliparous women is 5%, increasing to 10% with one child and 20% of women with 5 children.

b False
Stress incontinence can be helped by pelvic floor exercises if the incontinence is mild and the exercises are continued for several months. Terodolin is used in the treatment of detrusor instability. Surgery is effective provided urge incontinence does not co-exist.

c True
This is the basis of the Bonney test. Two fingers are inserted into the vagina along the anterior vaginal wall to support the urethro-vesical junction retropubically. The woman is asked to cough, and if incontinence is prevented it was presumed to be due to genuine stress incontinence. However, it has now been shown that this manoeuvre simply occludes the urethra and will prevent leakage of urine whatever the cause. It is therefore of no practical use.

d False
Up to 20% of all women over 18 years of age have either stress or urge incontinence at some time in their life, although many will not volunteer this information. History and examination alone may not be diagnostic, and urodynamic studies should be considered.

e False
The only large controlled study into postnatal exercises has failed to show any difference in subsequent incontinence ratios; however, these women have a lower incidence of pelvic pain and depression.

B20 a True
If either partner has evidence of warts, a sheath should be used during sexual intercourse and the affected partner treated. Venereal warts or condylomata accuminata are caused by the human papilloma viruses (HPVs).

b False
During pregnancy they may be large and fusiform.

c False
Podophylline is teratogenic when used locally. It can cause damage to the central nervous system and fetal death. It is, however, safe to use a 20% concentration, applied to the warts and washed off 6 hours later. It is extremely irritant to normal skin, and vasoline should be used to protect the surrounding area.

d True
There is increasing evidence of a correlation between condylomata accuminata and vulval cancer as well as cervical cancer. Certain strains of the HPV have been implicated, although other factors are undoubtedly involved.

e True
Vulval warts are thought to cause the rare, juvenile laryngeal papillomas in neonates.

B21 a False
A full blood count will not help the GP in his investigation and management of pruritus vulvae. The commonest causes of pruritus vulvae include atrophic vaginitis, infections and reactions to chemicals.

b True
To help exclude diabetes mellitus. Monilial infection (thrush) is frequently found in women with diabetes.

c True
Multiple biopsies may be needed to exclude carcinoma-in-situ of the vulva. Other white lesions seen on the vulva which are benign include vitiligo, hyperkeratosis, chronic papillomatous lesions and lichen sclerosis. Lichen sclerosis is not a predisposing factor for carcinoma of the vulva.

d True
Psoriasis of the vulva is uncommon. It can present classically as round lesions with linear excoriations, or as a non-specific rash. Psoriasis elsewhere on the body should be looked for. Local hydrocortisone cream and elimination of irritants are the advised treatment.

e True
This will help to diagnose vulval and vaginal infections. Common organisms implicated include *Trichomonas vaginalis*, *Candida albicans* and *Gardnerella*.

B22 a True

This is only useful in hypothalamic anovulation in women with a low body mass index, e.g. women with anorexia nervosa, malnourished or athletic women. Interestingly, a good nutritional status appears to be necessary for any successful treatment of anovulation. It has been reported that resumption of ovulation has occurred in obese women who have lost weight. The body mass index equals the weight in kilograms divided by the square of the height in metres^2.

b False

Danazol is an androgen and suppresses LH, FSH, oestrogen and progesterone. It therefore produces anovulation and amenorrhoea. It is indicated for endometriosis and fibrocystic breast disease.

c True

Clomiphene is an anti-oestrogen which blocks oestrogen receptors at hypothalamic and pituitary levels, preventing the negative feedback. As a consequence of this, FSH is released. Before starting on clomiphene, the GP must exclude nutritional problems and pituitary and ovarian failure. Clinically, this involves checking the body mass index and looking for evidence of oestrogen activity or ovarian failure. Blood tests should include serum FSH to exclude ovarian failure, and serum prolactin to exclude a prolactinoma.

d False

Pergonal is human gonadotrophin and is useful in the treatment of anovulatory patients. However, because of its side effects of hyperstimulation of the ovaries and subsequent multiple pregnancy, its use should be restricted to hospital specialists.

e False

Although bromocriptine is used in the treatment of hyperprolactinaemia, this should only be done after specialist endocrine assessment. This is to establish the cause of hyperprolactinoma and exclude a pituitary tumour.

B23 a True

Vaginal examination may help to find the following causes of primary amenorrhoea: cryptomenorrhoea, absent vagina and testicular feminisation. In cryptomenorrhoea, an imperforate hymen stops menstrual loss. A bluish membrane can be seen at the introitus, and treatment is by incision of this membrane. Absent vagina is important to diagnose, so that surgery can be considered early. There may be associated renal and skeletal abnormalities and these should also be looked for. In the testicular feminisation syndrome, the genotype is XY (male) but the phenotype (the outward appearance) is female. On vaginal examination, the vagina may be small and there is no uterus. Inguinal herniae may be found. Testes will be present and should be removed because of the risk of malignant change.

b True
However, investigation should be started. The GP should check weight, height and presence of secondary sexual characteristics. Laboratory tests that would be useful include serum prolactin, FSH, LH, progesterone, oestrogen and testosterone. An early specialist referral is important. Amenorrhoea should be investigated in 14-year-old girls who have failed to develop secondary sexual characteristics, and in 16-year-olds who have developed them.

c True
Measurement of FSH and LH helps to determine at which level the cause of amenorrhoea lies, i.e. outflow tract, ovary, anterior pituitary or hypothalamus.

d False
This is only done if a pituitary tumour is suspected, i.e. the serum prolactin is raised. Approximately one-third of women with secondary amenorrhoea will have a pituitary adenoma. X-ray may show erosion of the clinoid processes or enlargement of the pituitary fossa, with or without a double floor. CT scanning has now become a routine investigation to assess the pituitary fossa.

e True
However, this is unlikely to be available to most GPs, and the girl should be referred.

B24 a False
Rhesus haemolytic disease still occurs, mainly due to avoidable factors. It occurs when a rhesus D-negative woman, who has previously been exposed to the D antigen, has a rhesus D-positive child. Previous exposure may be due to an earlier pregnancy or a blood transfusion. However, it is now clear that this sensitisation can occur during an apparently normal first pregnancy. It seems likely that soon all rhesus-negative primigravida will be given anti-D at 28 and 34 weeks. The main problem is the supply of anti-D. IgG anti-D (100 μg) must be given to all rhesus D-negative women after delivering rhesus D-positive babies. The GP and the community midwife should check that the anti-D has been given by the hospital. The GP should also have access for anti-D (50 μg) to be given following spontaneous abortion.

b False
Detection of antibodies indicates that rhesus iso-immunisation has occurred. The importance of the antibodies is that the level relates reasonably well to the severity of the haemolytic disease in the fetus. However, it does not give enough precision to judge the optimal time for intervention. Investigation is now by obtaining a fetal blood sample for estimation of haemoglobin and antibody levels under ultrasound control. This is carried out only in highly specialised units, to which all such women should be referred.

c True
Transplacental haemorrhage may occur with threatened abortion, placental abruption, amniocentesis, chorionic villous sampling, fetoscopy and external cephalic version. Excluding those women known to have had a blood transfusion, anti-D antibodies have been found to develop in up to 2% of first pregnancies.

d True
Intra-uterine transfusion of rhesus-negative blood is given to reduce the haemolysis and its effects. This may allow the fetus to mature further before an early elective delivery.

e False
Unfortunately, this worsens in severity with each subsequent rhesus D-positive fetus.

B25 a True
This pain will be characteristically 14 days before menstruation and mid-cycle (Mittelschmerz). The pain will be helped by inhibiting ovulation with the combined oral contraceptive pill, which can be used providing the woman does not smoke and there are no other contraindications to its use.

b True
It is important to ask specifically about bowel symptoms and consider treatment in the presence of non-gynaecological symptoms. Treatment consists of dietary fibre manipulation, antispasmodics and a sympathetic doctor.

c True
Ectopic pregnancy should not be forgotten in any woman of reproductive age who complains of pelvic pain, even if the woman has been sterilised or her partner has had a vasectomy. Vaginal bleeding does not exclude an ectopic. Other symptoms, not always present, include amenorrhoea, a feeling of faintness and shoulder tip pain.

d True
Other symptoms that may be present are menorrhagia, deep dyspareunia, pelvic pain between menses and infertility. Rare symptoms include haematuria and rectal bleeding.

e True
An important cause of acute abdominal pain, predominantly in the right iliac fossa following an initial stage of poorly localised central abdominal pain.

B26 a True

Other possible causes, such as UTI, ovarian cyst, appendicitis, diabetes and raised intracranial pressure, should be excluded before diagnosing vomiting due to pregnancy (hyperemesis gravidarum). If the vomiting is severe, promethazine or prochlorperazine are used. This condition is more common with multiple pregnancy and with a hydatidiform mole. There is no evidence that hyperemesis is related to an increased risk of congenital abnormality.

b True

Urinary tract infections are generally much more common in pregnancy, due to ureteric dilatation and stasis, particularly in late pregnancy. Asymptomatic bacteriuria is more common in pregnancy and predisposes to pyelonephritis. An MSU should therefore be checked in every woman presenting with vomiting in pregnancy.

c True

This is characterised by sudden onset of severe abdominal pain and vomiting. A pelvic mass is usually palpable, but may be obscured by pain. A high index of suspicion is required, and if there is any doubt an ultrasound examination will be required.

d True

Although degenerating fibroids tend to present late in the pregnancy when the uterus is larger.

e False

Pre-eclampsia does not present before 20 weeks of pregnancy. It should be screened for from 20 weeks onwards. A strict definition of pre-eclampsia is difficult, but it has been described as a pregnancy-specific syndrome which may terminate in eclampsia (convulsions), and is characterised by hypertension and proteinuria.

B27 a False

Procidentia is the prolapse of the entire uterus through the introitus. Ulceration may occur, so it should be reduced as soon as possible and held in position by a pessary. Oestrogen cream will help to heal any ulceration that has occurred. All patients, except the very elderly, should be referred to a gynaecologist.

b True

It often is. The symptoms produced include the feeling of 'a lump coming down', stress incontinence, difficulty in defaecation and discharge from a procidenta. Backache is rarely caused by the prolapse, if it were it would be relieved by lying down.

c False
Operative management is the best treatment in all women with prolapse who are fit for anaesthetic. A *cystocoele*, prolapse of the upper two-thirds of the anterior vaginal wall, is corrected by an anterior repair (colporrhaphy) and a *rectocoele*, prolapse of the rectum and posterior wall of the vagina, is treated by a posterior repair (colpoperineorrhaphy). The other types of prolapse are *urethrocoeles*, a prolapse of the lower one-third of the anterior vaginal wall, and *enterocoeles*, a hernia of the pouch of Douglas into the posterior vaginal fornix. A Manchester repair is used for vault prolapse when preservation of the uterus is desired. More commonly, vaginal hysterectomy and repair are performed.

d True
This is uncommon and may be caused by a large cystocoele. Women presenting with urinary retention need a full pelvic examination and neurological assessment.

e False
There is no firm evidence that more liberal use of episiotomy is protective against stress incontinence, although it is associated with a lower frequency of anterior vaginal and labial tears.

B28 a False
Provided there are none of the usual contraindications the combined oral contraceptive pill is acceptable, but only after the HCG levels have returned to normal. This is the advice from Charing Cross Hospital, although other authorities have shown that it can be used before the HCG is back to normal.

b True
Women should be followed up by specialist centres, e.g. Charing Cross by regular serum beta-HCG and then urinary HCG. It is strongly advised that the woman does not become pregnant until 6 months after the HCG has returned to normal. Effective contraception is necessary. Clinically, a hydatidiform mole presents as a large-for-dates uterus, although this is not invariable, and vaginal bleeding. It is confirmed by an ultrasound scan. Following evacuation of a hydatidiform mole, 3% of women develop choriocarcinoma and another 15% have persistent mole. The incidence is increased in Eurasian and Chinese women, but it is uncommon in women of Afro-Caribbean descent.

c False
The risk is about 1 in 150 subsequent pregnancies, or a 10-fold risk compared to non-affected women.

d False
Most women will have a normal delivery after a hydatidiform mole. There is no increase in the incidence of prematurity, stillbirths or congenital malformations.

e False
Uterine perforation following evacuation is a possibility and is an important complication. A persistently high serum beta-HCG level, together with uterine pain and tenderness, suggest this complication may have occurred.

B29 a True
The annual mortality is 2000 deaths per year, with 4000 cases reported per year. This has remained unchanged since 1968. Organised screening programmes in British Columbia, Finland and Scotland have been followed by significant falls in mortality.

b True
Although cervical disease is still possible, it is extremely unlikely after the age of 65 if a woman has had at least 2 consecutive negative smears.

c True
There are a large number of minor abnormalities which cause considerable concern for the woman involved, and sympathetic counselling is essential. The most common of these minor abnormalities is cervical intra-epithelial neoplasia I (CIN I). In these cases, sexually transmitted disease should be looked for and treated, and the smear repeated in 6 months. More serious abnormalities are CIN II (moderate dysplasia), CIN III (severe dysplasia/carcinoma-in-situ) and invasive carcinoma.

d True
GPs in the UK are paid a percentage of the higher target depending on the percentage of smears actually performed in their practice. The lower payment is for 50–79% of women in this group. The smears must be adequate and not heavily bloodstained.

e False
Days 10–20 of the 28-day cycle are the optimum time for taking a smear which has few polymorphs and mature endocervical cells. From day 21 onwards, there is an increase in polymorphs which give a dirty background to the smear. Taking a smear during menstruation can also obscure the endocervical cells. However, with high-risk patients a smear should be taken when the opportunity arises.

B30 a True
The UK figures used to include all deaths whether caused by the pregnancy or not within one year of delivery or abortion. However the definition now excludes deaths more than 42 days after delivery.

b True
This figure has been falling slowly over recent years, but could probably still be reduced further. Indirect deaths will not be affected by obstetric care.

c True
Other common causes are pulmonary embolus and anaesthesia.

d True
There is a clear pattern of increased death due to this cause in older multiparous women, particularly if obese and delivered by caesarean section. It may be advisable to consider prophylaxis in such women.

e True
Although the numbers are small, this has implications for a rising caesarean section rate. However, it should be noted that some of these women would have other problems, such as severe hypertension.

B31 a True
A retroverted uterus is usually a normal variant, prevalent in up to 20% of normal women. It may be a sequela of pelvic pathology, including endometriosis and pelvic inflammatory disease, through scarring of the uterine support ligaments.

b False
If dyspareunia is found with a retroverted uterus, it is either incidental or related to endometriosis or pelvic inflammatory disease.

c False
Most retroverted uteruses will become axial or anteverted as the pregnant uterus rises out of the pelvis after 12 weeks. Incarceration used to be a problem 50 years ago, due to flattening of the pelvic brim as a result of rickets. If this rare event occurs, the woman will complain of urinary retention. It is best treated by catheterisation, which allows the uterus to move out of the pelvis.

d True
This occurs as a result of scarring of the uterosacral ligaments.

e True
Although surgery is rarely indicated as a primary procedure, it is sometimes used if benefit has been obtained by achieving anteversion with a Hodge pessary.

B32 a False
However, mosaicism XO/XX may occur. The somatic features of Turner's syndrome include slightly low birthweight, short stature, webbed neck, lymphoedema of the hands and feet and coarctation of the aorta. The ovaries are either absent or rudimentary ('streak' ovaries).

b False
Klinefelter's syndrome usually has a XXY karyotype and presents in adolescence. There is decreased libido, gynecomastia, small, firm testes and a wide arm span. The affected males are subfertile, mentally subnormal and may manifest antisocial tendencies.

c True
The majority of cases of Down's syndrome are due to non-dysjunction, which causes trisomy 21 with karyotype 47XX or 47XY. However, 3% of Down's syndrome have the karyotype 46XX or 46XY, and are due to translocation. This occurs if one of the parents has a balanced translocation, i.e. an intact chromosome (21) and another mixed chromosome (14), which contains material from chromosome 21. After union with a normal gamete, the conceptus will have 3 parts of chromosome 21. This cause of Down's syndrome is unrelated to maternal age. If the father carries the translocation, the risk of an affected child is 10%, but if the mother carries it the risk rises to 50%. Non-dysjunction, which causes most cases of Down's syndrome, increases in incidence with increasing maternal age. During meiosis there is non-dysjunction so that one gamete has an extra chromosome. During fertilisation, trisomy is produced by the union of this abnormal gamete with a normal gamete. 50% of these conceptuses will spontaneously abort. The other cause of Down's syndrome is mosaicism; in this, trisomy may develop during the early stages of division so that some of the cells have trisomy and some are normal, 46XX/47XX or 46XY/47XY.

d True
Treacher Collins' syndrome is a rare autosomal dominant condition. Affected individuals have oblique palpebral fissures, and flattened malar bones with an absent zygoma. If there is associated underdevelopment of the lower part of the face with absence of the outer ear and atresia of the internal auditory meati, the combination of appearances is known as Franceschetti's syndrome.

e True
Marfan's syndrome is inherited as an autosomal dominant. It affects the skeleton, the cardiovascular system and the eyes. The extremities are long with spidery fingers (arachnodactyly) and the palate is high arched. Aortic incompetence and aortic dissection occur, as well as mitral valve prolapse. Characteristically, upward dislocation of the lens occurs. Aortic dilatation and dissection are the main causes of premature death in this syndrome.

B33 a True
Down's syndrome is associated with ligamentous laxity which leads to both atlanto-axial subluxation and posterior atlanto-occipital subluxation. Flexion and extension views of the cervical spine should be obtained in Down's patients prior to any vigorous sporting activity. Down's is also associated with premature degenerative disease of the cervical spine.

b False
About 50% of Down's children have a single palmar crease. Other clinical features are: a round, flat face with upslanting palpebral fissures and epicanthic folds, broad hands with short fingers and an incurving little finger (clinodactyly), redundant skin over the nape of the neck and hypotonia at birth. Strabismus, nystagmus and myopia are common, as are malformed auricles, and a protruding tongue.

c False
Brushfield's spots (peripheral silver specks in the iris) are seen in about 50% of children with Down's syndrome. Koplik's spots are a feature of measles.

d True
Acute myeloblastic leukaemia in the newborn, and lymphoblastic leukaemia in older children are both relatively frequent in Down's syndrome, but transient leukaemoid reactions also occur. Together they affect 1% of all cases of Down's syndrome.

e True
The incidence of congenital heart disease in Down's syndrome is 40–70%. The most common abnormalities are AV canal defects (endocardial cushion defects), VSD and ASD. However, almost all forms of congenital cardiac malformation have been described, including tetralogy of Fallot. Down's syndrome is also associated with various gastrointestinal abnormalities, including duodenal stenosis and atresia, tracheo-oesophageal fistula, umbilical hernia, imperforate anus and Hirschsprung's disease.

B34 a True
High-dose oxygen should be given after the pharynx has been sucked out and the neonate has been laid on its side until fitting stops. If fitting continues, rectal valium should be given (0.25 mg/kg).

b True
It is essential that the serum glucose is measured. Hypoglycaemia is a common cause of neonatal fits. If the value is less than 1.4 mmol/l, hypoglycaemia may be present. A blood sample should be taken for glucose and calcium. If hypoglycaemia is suspected, 2–4 ml of 20% glucose per kg should be given slowly. When the fitting has stopped, continuous intragastric milk should be given.

c False
Hypothermia must be excluded. This exists if the rectal temperature is less than 35°C. It affects low birthweight infants paricularly, and can be easily prevented by covering the baby. The advice given is different in febrile convulsions occurring between the ages of 1 and 5 years, when hyperthermia is a considerable problem. Other causes of neonatal convulsions include hypoglycaemia, hypocalcaemia, asphyxia, meningitis and cerebral oedema.

d True
Hypoglycaemia, hypocalcaemia and meningitis all need urgent
exclusion. The neonate should be nursed and observed in an
incubator.

e False
In the neonate, *E.coli* and other Gram-negative organisms are the
most common causes. Treatment should be started with an
aminoglycoside (e.g. netilmicin) and penicillin until the causative
organism is isolated. In children, meningococcus is an important
cause of meningitis. In any child seen at home with suspected
meningitis, a single intramuscular (or slow intravenous) injection
of 20–40 mg/kg of penicillin should be given by the GP.

B35 a True
Uterine rupture can cause severe maternal shock as well as
abdominal pain and vaginal bleeding. Half the cases occur in
women with a uterine scar. Other risk factors include internal
podalic version, oxytocin administration in women with high
parity, and difficult forceps delivery. GP trainees doing obstetrics
should not start oxytocin infusions without discussion with senior
colleagues.

b True
Although rare (1 in 81 000 deliveries), this complication has a
mortality of 86%. It is associated with older women and high parity.
The clinical features include extreme shock with cyanosis,
followed by intractable uterine bleeding. The woman should be
resuscitated and transferred to an intensive care unit.

c True
Massive pulmonary embolism causes severe chest pain, dyspnoea
and collapse. The woman will be cyanosed, tachypnoeic and have
a raised jugular venous pressure. The at-risk patients are: those
who have a caesarean section (10 times higher), older women,
multiparity, obesity (1 in 5 deaths due to PE are in women over
76 kg), hospitalised women, introduction of the combined oral
contraceptive pill before 6 weeks post delivery, previous PE or
thrombosis, and SLE or other thrombotic diseases.

d True
A reaction may occur and cause severe shock. It remains important
to check all blood before it is given to a woman, to ensure that
mistakes are not made.

e True
The shock is usually neurogenic in origin, from traction on the
round ligaments, but can be complicated by haemorrhage from the
placental site. It is best treated by replacement of the uterus and
resuscitation with i.v. fluids. An i.v. oxytocic agent should be given.
The uterus can be replaced hydrostatically with warm saline.
Uterine inversion is best prevented by applying traction on the cord
while the uterus is contracted.

B36 a True

This is the claim form for medical services and should be signed by the patient at booking with the GP. It is forwarded to the FPC after the post-partum examination at 6 weeks. The 6-week check is popular with mothers, and allows them an opportunity to discuss their concerns about the birth and future pregnancies. Complications from the birth can be followed up and the infant examined. Registration of the baby in the practice should be checked. It also allows the GP to assess the maternity services the practice offers, and continue the relationship he/she has developed with the family.

b False

If the woman is symptomatic (e.g. vulval pain, dyspareunia) then a vaginal examination should be suggested to her. Otherwise, vaginal examination does not need to be performed.

c True

If the maternal BP has not returned to normal, the pre-eclampsia may have revealed chronic renal disease or pre-existing hypertension. The mother must be investigated further and appropriate treatment started.

d False

Pregnancy may have occurred, especially in non-lactating women. If there is doubt about pregnancy, insertion of the coil should be delayed until the next menses.

e False

Although interpretation can be more difficult than in the non-puerperium.

B37 a True

Cardiotocographs (CTG) are a screening test and an indirect method of assessing the fetus. Direct assessment by fetal pH should be considered before any operative delivery for fetal distress.

b True

A pH of 7.25 is within the normal range. However, it must be interpreted in the light of all the other features of the labour. Furthermore it should be repeated if any CTG abnormality recurs, as the level can easily fall. The pH drops as more lactic acid is produced by anaerobic pathways secondary to hypoxia. At a pH of less than 7.2, immediate delivery should be expedited. Between 7.2 and 7.25, the test should be repeated 30 minutes later. Despite this, however, there is a poor correlation between cord pH levels and subsequent handicap.

c False
Although some operators prefer this position, many women do not like it. Care must be taken in the lithotomy position that the woman is not flat, as the gravid uterus may obstruct the IVC, causing maternal hypotension and further fetal distress. A suitable alternative is the left lateral position. The method of obtaining a sample involves visualisation of the fetal head through an amnioscope. The smaller the amount of cervical dilatation, the more difficult the procedure. The exposed part of the fetal head is cleaned and then ethyl chloride spray is used to induce hyperaemia. Gel is then smeared over the skin so that when the blood is obtained it tends to form globules.

d False
This will give a false reading. Care must be taken with good technique to ensure that only fetal blood, not liquor or maternal blood, is aspirated.

e False
However, care must be taken to ascertain the fetal part from which the blood will be taken.

B38 a True
Placenta accreta is, fortunately, rare. It is the morbid adherence of the placenta to the uterine wall. If the woman wants further children, a conservative approach with oxytocins or prostaglandins can be tried, provided the bleeding is minimal. Otherwise, hysterectomy is necessary.

b False
There is a high risk of primary postpartum haemorrhage and sepsis. However, if the placenta is left 60 minutes after delivery, 50% of women will not need a manual removal. It is best avoided with skilled management of the third stage.

c True
Therefore an intravenous cannula must be positioned and blood sent for cross-matching. The woman must be resuscitated prior to delivery of the placenta. A repeat dose of i.v. syntometrine should be given.

d False
50% will deliver at 60 minutes if blood loss is low. The remainder will be delivered after manual evacuation, the rare exception being placenta accreta which may require hysterectomy. Manual removal carries the danger of uterine rupture and must be performed with the operator's hand controlling the uterine fundus abdominally. A course of antibiotics is usually given to prevent infection following this procedure. Occasionally, a woman may be encountered who has had a hysterotomy, an outdated operation for aborting second trimester fetuses. This is important to know, as she is at risk of uterine rupture during pregnancy and labour.

e True
The incidence of placenta accreta increases considerably.

B39 a True
Instrumental deliveries are increased. Some of the factors involved may be poor timing of top-up doses, and anxiety about the length of the second stage. This is often prolonged, but as the woman has less fatigue and acidosis there is less fetal acidosis. The quality of pain control should allow for easy instrumental delivery.

b True
For this reason, it is essential that the woman has an intravenous infusion of Hartmann's solution in place before the epidural is performed. If the blood pressure drops by more than 20 mmHg, the infusion should be speeded up. If this has no effect, then ephedrine 5 mg is given.

c False
Urinary retention occurs and the woman must be catheterised intermittently. For the first stage of labour the block covers the nerves T10–L1, while for the second stage S2–S5 are covered.

d False
If the epidural needle punctures the dura, up to 70% of women will get headaches. This can be treated with Hartmann's epidural solution via a bacterial filter. The woman should be kept flat and started on a laxative to prevent straining during defaecation. A blood patch may be required in refractory cases.

e False
However, there is some reduction in the pelvic floor tone which may reduce the ability of the presenting part to rotate correctly.

B40 a False
Diabetes is a well-recognised cause of large-for-dates babies. How much of this macrosomia can be prevented by good diabetic control is unclear. If pre-eclampsia develops, intra-uterine growth retardation can occur and the baby can then be small for dates. This is uncommon, and the perinatal mortality high.

b False
The mean birthweight at 42 weeks is greater than at 40 weeks. Babies who are small for gestational age at 42 weeks have increased morbidity from asphyxia and meconium aspiration.

c True
Pre-eclampsia is a common cause of small-for-dates babies. The pathophysiology of asymmetrical intra-uterine growth retardation is thought to be the same whether pre-eclampsia occurs or not.

d True
Smoking causes a small reduction in the mean birthweight. However, it may be associated with an increase in perinatal mortality.

e False
There is no data to support this, although many think there is a link.
There may also be an increase in the risk of pre-term delivery.

5. Paper C

C1 Hypertension in pregnancy:
   a Maternal outcome correlates with mean systolic pressure
   b Requires proteinuria for a diagnosis of pre-eclampsia
   c Can be treated by anti-hypertensive drugs to reduce subsequent pre-eclampsia
   d Requires induction at 38 weeks
   e May be familial

C2 Vitamin K:
   a Is ineffective in pre-term infants so should not be given routinely
   b May not be needed in bottle-fed neonates
   c Prevents osteomalacia
   d Should be given routinely to epileptic women who are taking anticonvulsants in the third trimester
   e Is used if over-anticoagulation occurs in a pregnant woman having heparin therapy for a deep vein thrombosis

C3 Uterine fibroids:
   a Can undergo malignant change
   b Are more common in parous women
   c Are predominantly submucosal
   d May undergo degeneration during pregnancy
   e May cause infertility

C4 Congenital abnormalities:
   a Affect 2% of all deliveries
   b Are commoner in marriages between cousins
   c Account for 20% of first week deaths
   d Are commoner in twin pregnancies
   e May be caused by Cytomegalovirus infection

C5 Smoking during pregnancy:
   a Increases risk of low birthweight babies
   b Increases risk of perinatal death
   c Increases risk of pre-term delivery
   d Increases risk of impaired reading ability of the offspring
   e Increases risk of pre-eclampsia

C6   Blood tests at booking should include:
   a   Hepatitis B surface antigen
   b   Cytomegalovirus antibodies
   c   Consort's blood group in Rhesus-negative mothers
   d   Haemoglobin electrophoresis in Pakistani women
   e   *Treponema pallidum* haemagglutination antibodies

C7   Which of the following are true of postpartum hypertension?:
   a   Mean arterial pressure progressively rises during the first 5 days after delivery
   b   Symptoms and signs may appear for the first time postpartum
   c   Does not need treatment
   d   Cannot cause maternal death
   e   Treatment is likely to be needed for at least 6 months after delivery

C8   Concerning screening for ovarian cancer:
   a   Using serum monoclonal antibody CA 125 fits Wilson's criteria for screening
   b   Using colour flow Doppler fits Wilson's criteria for screening
   c   Ultrasound screening is cost effective and of clinical benefit
   d   Ultrasound screening may result in unnecessary laparotomies
   e   Ultrasound screening reduces mortality from the disease

C9   Jaundice in pregnancy:
   a   May be a terminal event in pre-eclampsia
   b   When due to acute hepatitis usually causes abortion or stillbirth
   c   With pruritus and raised alkaline phosphatase, is generally benign
   d   May follow severe hyperemesis gravidarum
   e   With acute fatty liver is associated with markedly abnormal liver function tests

C10   Pregnant women who are opiate addicts:
   a   Should be tested for HIV infection
   b   Have an increased risk of pre-term delivery
   c   Should stop opiates as soon as pregnancy is confirmed
   d   Produce infants who experience withdrawal side-effects
   e   Will require more frequent doses of pethidine if used in labour

C11   The following may be associated with a lower Apgar score:
   a   Meconium staining of the liquor
   b   Tight nuchal cord
   c   Normal cord pH
   d   Pethidine use in labour
   e   General anaesthesia

C12 The following conditions are routinely screened for in newborn infants in the UK:
a Phenylketonuria
b Hypothyroidism
c Cystic fibrosis
d Tuberculosis
e Deafness

C13 The following may occur on a normal cervix:
a Nabothian cysts
b Columnar epithelium on the ectocervix
c Leukoplakia
d Contact bleeding
e Punctation

C14 Alcohol during pregnancy:
a Is safe if only 2 units are consumed per day
b Causes an increased rate of spontaneous abortion
c Causes symmetrical growth retardation
d Is a cause of microcephaly
e Causes hyperactivity behavioural disturbance in infants

C15 Analgesia in labour:
a Nitrous oxide and air inhalation rarely cause side-effects
b Pethidine increases the risk of gastric aspiration if a general anaesthetic is required
c A transcutaneous nerve stimulator (TNS) is useful for the second stage
d May be given as diamorphine
e Epidural analgesia increases the incidence of postpartum haemorrhage

C16 Postpartum pyrexia:
a The incidence is significantly increased with the use of internal fetal monitoring
b Occurs more frequently after vaginal delivery than after caesarean section
c Is usually caused by group A streptococcus
d Is predisposed to by delaying the rupture of membranes during labour
e May be caused by septic thrombophlebitis

C17 Ovarian cysts in pregnancy:
a Are functional in most cases
b If pathological are usually benign teratomas
c May obstruct delivery
d Are malignant in approximately 1 in 100 cysts removed
e May be aspirated under ultrasound control if unilocular

C18 Eclampsia:
a Usually occurs antenatally
b Is now preventable in all cases
c Is commonly treated with magnesium sulphate in the UK
d Should be treated with intravenous phenytoin
e Is prevented by low dose aspirin

C19 Puerperal psychosis:
a Is usually manic in type
b Requires admission to hospital in approximately 1 in 1000 births
c Should be treated by separation of the baby from the mother for its protection
d Has an increased risk of suicide
e Is often recurrent

C20 Dyspareunia:
a Post delivery, is usually psychosomatic
b Usually has an organic cause if only present on deep penetration
c Is common after posterior repair
d May be due to endometriosis
e Should be referred for psychosexual counselling only as a last resort

C21 The following situations require referral by the GP for colposcopy:
a A borderline smear
b A persistent inflammatory smear
c A cervical polyp
d Post-coital bleeding
e Post-menopausal bleeding

C22 Vomiting in the first 24 hours of life may be due to:
a Meconium in the stomach
b Diaphragmatic hernia
c Meningitis
d Necrotising enterocolitis
e Hydrocephalus

C23 If a woman does not wish to breastfeed, which of the following methods helps to reduce lactation safely?
a Fluid restriction
b Breast binding
c Bromocriptine
d Stilboestrol
e The combined oral contraceptive pill

C24 Which of the following changes normally occur at birth in the fetus?:

    a Complete closure of the ductus arteriosus
    b Collapse of the ductus venosus
    c Pulmonary vascular resistance increases
    d Anatomical closure of the foramen ovale
    e Loss of heat due to evaporation of amniotic fluid

C25 Cephalopelvic disproportion:

    a Can be diagnosed antenatally
    b Is a contraindication to oxytocin in a primigravida
    c Should be treated with oxytocin in parous women
    d In the UK, is most commonly due to nutritional factors
    e Can be treated by forceps under general anaesthesia

C26 The following are associated with spontaneous miscarriage:

    a Diethylstilboestrol exposure in utero
    b Previous prostaglandin termination
    c Increasing maternal age
    d Smoking
    e Working with a VDU screen

C27 Twin pregnancies:

    a Always arise from two ova
    b Are commoner in women over 35
    c Have an increased risk of pre-eclampsia
    d Women should be routinely admitted for bed rest
    e The perinatal mortality rate is similar to that for singleton pregnancy

C28 A healthy pregnant woman:

    a Requires calcium supplements if she originates from the Indian subcontinent
    b Needs an extra 300 kcal per day
    c Should reduce exercise to conserve energy
    d Requires iron supplementation
    e Requires extra vitamin B complex

C29 In a normal first pregnancy:

    a An ultrasound scan should be performed at 32 weeks to assess fetal growth
    b Pelvic examination should be performed at 36 weeks to assess the pelvic capacity
    c The head should be engaged at 38 weeks
    d The woman should be seen weekly in a consultant unit from 36 weeks
    e The Domino delivery arrangement is not allowed

C30 Perinatal mortality in the UK:
 a Has been reduced by the more liberal use of caesarean section
 b Includes babies over 500 g in weight
 c Shows little geographical variation
 d Is due to congenital malformation in 25% of cases
 e Includes deaths occurring in the first month

C31 Sexual dysfunction:
 a May be due to depression
 b May be due to the treatment of depression
 c Commonly occurs after hysterectomy
 d May result in vaginismus
 e May be successfully treated by a psychologist

C32 Endometrial cancer:
 a Multiparous women are three times more likely to develop it than nulliparous women
 b Commonly causes enlargement of the uterus
 c May be treated by hysterectomy only
 d Advanced cases can be treated with high dose progesterone
 e Affects postmenopausal and menstruating women equally

C33 Cancer of the vulva:
 a Shows ulceration late in the disease
 b May be treated by simple vulvectomy in early cases
 c Is radiosensitive
 d Accounts for 5% of gynaecological cancers
 e Initially spreads by the blood stream

C34 Anorexia nervosa:
 a Has a mortality of 30%
 b Causes amenorrhoea
 c Has an increased incidence in siblings of an affected person
 d Patients usually require vitamin supplements
 e Causes breast atrophy

C35 Ovulation:
 a Occurs 72 hours after the LH surge
 b Can be confirmed by day 21 progesterone estimation
 c Occurs 14 days before menstruation
 d After childbirth, can occur before the first period
 e Has occurred if Spinnbarkheit is demonstrated

C36 Which of the following antibiotics reduce the efficiency of the oral contraceptive pill?:
- **a** Amoxycillin
- **b** Cephradine
- **c** Ampicillin
- **d** Tetracycline
- **e** Trimethoprim

C37 Hysterectomy:
- **a** Has less morbidity if performed vaginally
- **b** Removal of the ovaries should be discussed over the age of 45
- **c** Is the treatment of choice for CIN 3 once childbearing is complete
- **d** May affect bladder function
- **e** Has an operative mortality of approximately 1 in 2000

C38 Gonococcal infection:
- **a** Infects the cervix
- **b** May involve the Bartholin's gland
- **c** May present with a rash and arthritis
- **d** Crosses the placenta
- **e** Is commonly confirmed by serology

C39 Concerning inflammatory bowel disease in women:
- **a** The condition is more likely to relapse during pregnancy
- **b** It is a recognised cause of infertility
- **c** Salazopyrine is safe to use during pregnancy
- **d** It can cause a macrocytic blood picture
- **e** Surgery should be avoided during pregnancy

C40 The contraceptive diaphragm:
- **a** Is usually a cervical cap
- **b** Protects against cervical neoplasia
- **c** Requires re-fitting after a caesarean section
- **d** Should be left in for a maximum of 3 hours after intercourse
- **e** Has a failure rate of 29 per 100 women years even in motivated women

6. Paper C Answers

C1 a True
Untreated severe hypertension causes death by cerebral haemorrhage.
b True
Although this may occur late in the disease process. Oedema is no longer required to make a diagnosis of pre-eclampsia.
c False
The evidence that pre-eclampsia is prevented by anti-hypertensive drugs in women undergoing essential hypertension treatment is weak.
d False
This may cause more problems than it solves, because the cervix may not be favourable and, hence, caesarean section becomes more likely.
e True
As may pre-eclampsia.

C2 a False
Parenteral vitamin K (1 mg) is less effective in pre-term infants due to liver immaturity. However, it does have some effect and should be given to prevent haemorrhagic disease of the newborn.
b True
The concentration of vitamin K in infant formula or cow's milk is considerably higher than in breast milk. Some units have now stopped administering vitamin K to healthy, formula-fed neonates.
c False
Vitamin D prevents osteomalacia. Vitamin K prevents haemorrhagic disease of the newborn. It is necessary for the synthesis of clotting factors II, VII, IX and X. Bleeding typically occurs in affected breast-fed babies between days 3 and 6 post-partum. The presenting factor is usually melaena or haematemesis, but it may present as haematuria or umbilical stump bleeding. If it occurs, vitamin K should be given. Signs of shock or repeated substantial bleeding should be treated with fresh frozen plasma.

d True
Anticonvulsants depress vitamin K dependent factors in the fetus. Oral vitamin K should be given to mothers from 32 weeks of pregnancy onwards. Parenteral vitamin K must be given to all neonates born to mothers who are treated epileptics.

e False
Stopping the heparin will usually correct the over-anticoagulation, as heparin has a short half-life. If rapid reversal is required, protamine sulphate is a specific antidote. Oral anticoagulants antagonise the effects of vitamin K, so vitamin K administration will correct over-anticoagulation due to warfarin.

C3   a True
This is extremely rare. Fibroids may undergo sarcomatous change, but this risk should not influence the management in most women.

b False
Fibroids (leiomyomas) are more common in nulliparous women and in women of Afro-Caribbean and Japanese descent. Incidence increases with increasing age.

c False
Only 10% are submucosal (under the endometrium). 70% are intramural, with the remaining 10% subserosal (under the peritoneum).

d True
'Red' degeneration may occur during pregnancy and can usually be treated expectantly with analgesics. However, surgical intervention is occasionally needed, and myomectomy can be performed but with some risk of labour.

e True
The submucosal type may cause infertility. Multiple fibroids or large fibroids may cause recurrent abortion. Myomectomy should be considered.

C4   a True
Although many of these abnormalities may be treatable, e.g. tracheo-oesophageal fistula.

b True
This is particularly true of autosomal recessive conditions. If the family history is negative, there is a 1 in 20 risk of an abnormal pregnancy, which is approximately double that of the normal population.

c False
Approximately one-third of first week deaths are due to congenital abnormality.

d True
This is almost certainly confined to monozygous twins and concordance (i.e. both twins affected) may be as high as 30% for abnormalities such as congenital dislocation of the hip. Other abnormalities have a higher incidence but lower rate of concordance, e.g. cardiac abnormalities and neural tube defects.

e True
Infection in utero with CMV causes many abnormalities, including microcephaly, deafness and hydrocephalus.

C5 a True
Women who smoke produce infants which are, on average, 170 g lighter, and the risk of having a baby with a birthweight under 2500 g is about twice that in non-smoking mothers. Apart from reduced birthweight, other adverse perinatal outcomes are more controversial. It is important to remember that, while smoking should be actively discouraged, a sympathetic approach should be used. 50% of women who smoke during pregnancy feel guilty, and not all bad outcomes of pregnancy can be blamed on smoking. The effects of passive smoking of the husband's cigarettes are not yet clear.

b True
Perinatal deaths are increased in smoking mothers. There is also an increased risk of spontaneous abortion. Research is not in agreement about the risk of fetal abnormality.

c True
Some women believe that the reduced length of pregnancy and the lower birthweight will ensure an easier labour. However, there is a delay in maturation of the fetus. Interestingly, 10% of women smoke more during pregnancy than they do normally.

d True
There are increased problems with reading and educational standards in general up to the age of 11 in children born to smoking mothers.

e False
There is a reduced incidence of pre-eclampsia in smokers, but the perinatal mortality is higher.

C6 a True
It has been shown not to be possible to identify all carriers of hepatitis B by screening only those at apparent risk, e.g. women from the Far East, tattooed women. All personnel delivering intra-partum care should be vaccinated against hepatitis B.

b False
Even if negative (40%), prevention of primary infection is not possible and hence screening has no practical value.

c False
If the woman becomes sensitised then it is worth checking her partner's genotype. The presence of maternal antibodies does not indicate whether or not the fetus carries the antigen. It is therefore helpful to determine whether the woman's partner is homozygous or heterozygous. If the partner is homozygous then the fetus will carry the antigen but if the partner is heterozygous the risk is 50%.

d True
If they are found to carry the trait, then their partners should also be tested. If both are positive, they have a 1 in 4 chance of having a baby with the disease and can be offered pre-natal diagnosis.

e False
Initial screening is by the VDRL (Venereal Disease Reference Laboratory). If positive, more sensitive tests such as the TPHA will be required.

C7   a True
Therefore it is important to monitor and record BP during this period. The rise is exaggerated in hypertensive women.

b True
Symptoms of headache and epigastric discomfort should be taken seriously.

c False
Treatment should be used so that severe hypertension can be avoided. Methyldopa is best avoided because of its side-effects of tiredness and depression. Nifedipine and labetalol can be used.

d False
A maternal death has been reported on the sixth post-partum day following a fit.

e False
Antihypertensive treatment can usually be stopped within 4 weeks after delivery. The BP should be checked after cessation of treatment to ensure it has remained at a normal level.

C8   a False
This is a research tool and has not been fully evaluated for a screening program. It appears that it will not contribute to the early diagnosis of ovarian cancer.

b False
Research has been undertaken using real-time ultrasound, colour flow Doppler and serum CA 125 to screen for ovarian cancer. None of these methods at present satisfies Wilson's screening criteria.

c False
It is highly expensive and creates a great deal of morbidity due to unnecessary surgery.

d True
Many ovarian masses suspected on ultrasound screening are benign and not likely to become malignant. In some cases, suspected masses are simply loops of normal bowel.

e False
This remains far from proven at the present time.

C9 a True
Although the liver is not primarily involved in pre-eclampsia or eclampsia, jaundice can occur. Other rare liver complications of pre-eclampsia include subcapsular haematoma, liver rupture and liver necrosis.

b False
Apart from the increase in pre-term deliveries (20%), acute non-fulminant hepatitis has very little effect on the pregnancy. However, acute liver failure can cause high maternal and perinatal mortality. Infants born to hepatitis B carriers should be protected at birth with both active and passive immunisation.

c True
Intrahepatic cholestasis in pregnancy has a good prognosis. It may present with pruritus or with signs of obstructive jaundice (pale stools, dark urine). The pruritus is treated with cholestyramine, and vitamin K is given intramuscularly to prevent deficiency and subsequent haemorrhage. Once delivery has occurred there is rapid return to normal. There is a family history in over 25% of cases and it tends to recur in subsequent pregnancies.

d True
Jaundice is uncommon and only occurs in very severe forms of hyperemesis gravidarum. It is thought to be due to severe protein and vitamin malnutrition.

e False
Mildly raised bilirubin and transaminase levels combined with a high uric acid are characteristic of acute fatty liver of pregnancy. The aetiology is uknown. It has a rapid onset in the third trimester, presenting with abdominal pain, vomiting and headache. The mother will be afebrile and jaundiced. Complications include encephalopathy, DIC, renal failure and death. The treatment involves hospitalisation, immediate delivery and supportive therapy for liver failure. There is high maternal and fetal mortality.

C10 a True
After appropriate counselling. If testing is refused, precautions should be taken as if they are HIV-positive to prevent spillage of blood and to protect staff.

b True
Although this may be a social class variable.

c False
Sudden cessation of opiates is not recommended. Heroin addicts are usually better on methadone.

d True
Withdrawal can develop within 6 hours of delivery. Infants of opiate addicts should be admitted to the neonatal unit.

e True
An epidural may be a more effective method of pain relief.

C11 a True
Although this is often due to the action taken to prevent aspiration.

b True
This is a relatively common cause of an unsuspected 'flat' baby. Since the insult is likely to have been short-lived, the infant invariably responds to resuscitation.

c True
Umbilical artery pH measures a metabolic response, whereas the Apgar score is a description of certain aspects of neonatal behaviour. It is therefore not surprising that one can be depressed and the other normal, and vice versa.

d True
It can contribute to a low Apgar score by its depressant effect on the neonate's respiratory effort. If required, it can be reversed by naloxone.

e True
Anaesthetic agents do cross the placenta, and although they may be metabolised quickly by the mother this is not always the case with the neonate.

C12 a True
Phenylketonuria is a rare condition occurring in about 1 in 10 000 births. After feeding has been established by the fifth day, a heel prick blood sample is collected. There is an enzyme defect in the disorder, resulting in high serum levels of phenylalanine which causes progressive cerebral dysfunction and severe mental defect. All positive results by heel-prick blood testing require further investigation. Treatment is dietary, with low phenylalanine milk substitutes. The disorder is autosomal recessive, as with most enzyme defects. Normal intellectual development can be achieved and the diet can be relaxed after brain growth is complete. If a woman with the disorder becomes pregnant, it is important that she reverts back to a strict low phenylalanine diet in order to avoid cerebral impairment in the fetus.

b True
The same heel prick blood is used to detect hypothyroidism. Thyroid stimulating hormone will be raised. Clinical features of hypothyroidism in the newborn may not be apparent until after the first month. Features include slowness to cry, dry skin, sluggish movements, low temperature and persistent mild jaundice. Thyroxine therapy should be started as soon as possible to avoid cretinism.

c False

There is no suitable screening test for cystic fibrosis. 15% of affected neonates will present with meconium ileus. Diagnosis is by the sweat test. Most will present in childhood with recurrent respiratory infections, steatorrhoea or poor growth.

d False

Neonatal tuberculosis is extremely rare in the UK. It can be acquired from the mother before or after birth. The diagnosis is usually made by chest X-ray, as the tuberculin test will be negative at this stage. Maternal tuberculosis is more common in certain groups, e.g. women of Asian descent, and routine BCG is given to these high risk groups.

e False

Hearing can be subjectively assessed by the mother. Any parental concerns, particularly at the six-week check, require further investigation. Objective assessment can be made with an acoustic cradle bed, but this is not readily available for mass screening.

C13 a True

Nabothian cysts are common and are a normal feature of the adult cervix. They are retention cysts of endocervical columnar cells covered by squamous metaplasia. They may vary in size from microscopic to macroscopic.

b True

The vagina is lined by squamous epithelium, and the cervix by columnar epithelium. The squamocolumnar junction lies on the endocervix but moves in a caudal direction as the cervix enlarges under the influence of oestrogen at the menarche and pregnancy, and with use of the contraceptive pill. Columnar epithelium is therefore visible at the external os.

c False

Leukoplakia describes a visible white area, which should be further investigated. Biopsy should be considered to exclude carcinoma-in-situ.

d True

Contact bleeding occurs after cervical trauma during the taking of a smear. It may be due to the presence of thin columnar epithelium, but if suspicious should be referred for colposcopy.

e False

This is a colposcopic term used to describe the stippled appearance of capillary vessels at an abnormal squamocolumnar junction (the transformation zone) usually after the application of acetic acid. It is suggestive of cervical intra-epithelial neoplasia.

C14 a False

No critical dose is known and the best advice is none at all. Binge drinking appears to have more detrimental effects on the fetus than a background consumption, particularly in the first trimester.

b True
It has been reported that there is double the risk even with as little as 2 units/week.

c True
Growth retardation is symmetrical. This is because the alcohol influences the developing fetus in the first trimester, rather than causing later malnutrition.

d True
The fetal alcohol syndrome describes the effects on the neonate caused by maternal alcohol consumption. There is a correlation between lower birthweight and a higher level of alcohol intake. The features of the syndrome include: microphthalmia, prominent epicanthic folds, short nose, thin upper lip and low-set ears. There may be developmental delay, neurological abnormalities and mental retardation.

e True
Generally small infants with low IQ and hyperactive behaviour who tend to make poor progress at school.

C15 a False
Nausea and vomiting occurs in at least 20% of women using inhalation analgesia during labour. There is also a potential risk of maternal mortality due to accidental overdosage resulting in aspiration of gastric contents. The main drawback is inadequate pain relief.

b True
Pethidine slows stomach emptying, and the anaesthetist will need to be informed if it has been given.

c False
It may be useful for early first stage, but it is not generally useful in the second stage.

d True
This is not widely used in labour in the UK but it is effective. It induces some degree of amnesia and so is useful for cases of stillbirth and termination where epidurals are not available.

e False
Epidural analgesia has no effect on the third stage of labour.

C16 a False
Studies have failed to show any increased risk of intra-uterine infection other than the risk identified with vaginal examination. Endometritis is doubled in women with premature rupture of the membranes who have 4 or more vaginal examinations, compared to those women who have 3 or less.

b False
The risk of infection is 10–20 times greater with caesarean section. There are various reasons for this, including blood at the wound site and increased bacterial invasion of the placental bed.

c False
The major epidemics of puerperal sepsis were caused by the group A streptococcus. This organism is now, however, a rare cause of infection. Group B streptococcus, *E.coli*, *Staphylococcus aureus*, *Bacteroides*, *Clostridium*, *Mycoplasma* and *Chlamydia trachomatis* have been found to be causative agents. Often, there is a mixed infection. Broad spectrum antibiotics should be used and started as soon as cervical and high vaginal swabs, an MSU and blood cultures have been taken.

d False
Rupturing the membranes removes the natural barrier to chorio-amnionitis and predisposes to neonatal and postpartum infection.

e True
This is an uncommon cause. Often, there are no specific clinical findings but it should be suspected in a woman with a high swinging fever, tachycardia and failure to respond to antibiotics. In addition to antibiotics, a trial of intravenous heparin should produce an improvement in 2 days.

C17 a True
Some degree of cystic change in the ovary is normal as it hypertrophies to maintain the pregnancy before the placenta can take over. Some of this cystic change may persist.

b True
Benign teratomas (dermoid cysts) are the commonest tumour found in pregnancy. If found, they should be removed as they commonly undergo torsion. The next most common type of cysts are the cystadenomas.

c True
They are a cause of a high head at term, and unstable lie. With the widespread use of ultrasound, most are found in the second trimester.

d True
Removal is indicated if the cyst is more than 8 cm in diameter or multilocular. Of these, at least 1% will prove to be malignant.

e True
The fluid is then sent to cytology to exclude any chance of malignancy.

C18 a False
Most cases now occur in the post natal period.

b False
Many women have few or no premonitory symptoms, and eclampsia can occur rapidly and despite anti-convulsants.

c False
There is no evidence that magnesium sulphate is an effective anti-convulsant agent, although it is commonly used in the USA for historic reasons. It does not cross the blood-brain barrier in significant amounts and has no effect on maternal blood pressure. Magnesium overdosage is possible and magnesium crosses the placenta.

d False
Intravenous diazepam is the drug of first choice for convulsions. Other action required is to maintain a clear airway and aspirate any vomit or secretions.

e False
Even though low dose aspirin may reduce the incidence of pre-eclampsia, those women that do still get it are going to run the risk of developing eclampsia.

C19 a False
Although the manic type of puerperal psychosis does occur, it is less common than the depressive type. The manic form is more difficult to identify because the women seem so rational, whereas severe depression is usually more obvious.

b True
Many hospital practitioners will not realise how common puerperal psychosis is, because it tends to occur after discharge from hospital.

c False
Special mother and baby units are available for the treatment of severe puerperal psychosis, and it is rarely necessary to separate them.

d True
This is a real risk, and such deaths will be included in the maternal mortality figures.

e True
The risk of a recurrence after a future pregnancy may be as high as 1 in 4. Prophylaxis with progesterone has been suggested but not scientifically evaluated, and a trial is at present underway to assess the value of prophylactic oestrogen therapy.

C20 a False
Most cases of dyspareunia at this stage revolve around the perineal trauma at delivery. Most will settle with time, and reassurance is usually the best therapy.

b True
Psychosexual causes tend to produce superficial dyspareunia, i.e. on initial penetration.

c True
If the woman is still sexually active, special care is required to achieve a satisfactory repair yet not narrow the vagina too much.

d True
Deposits of endometriosis on the utero-sacral ligaments are the cause of dyspareunia in this condition.

e False
A careful history and examination should be undertaken. If there is no local cause, then a laparoscopy may be indicated if endometriosis is suspected. Psychosexual problems are common, however, and appropriate referral should not be delayed.

C21 a False
Most cytology laboratories will advise repeating the smear after 6 months. If the smear remains borderline, referral should be considered.

b True
After the first inflammatory smear, swabs should be taken to exclude an infection. After appropriate treatment the smear should be repeated after 2 months. If it remains inflammatory, the woman should be referred for colposcopy. Colposcopy involves visualising the cervix under bright illumination with ×10–40 magnification. The cervix is inspected after removal of mucus and application of 5% acetic acid. Abnormal areas stain white. After visualisation biopsies are performed. It may be an unpleasant procedure for some women, and preparatory explanation by the referring doctor is important.

c False
Cervical polyps are usually avulsed and the base is cauterised if necessary. A D&C may also be indicated in older women, to exclude intra-uterine pathology.

d False
Suspected carcinoma requires a formal biopsy and so colposcopy may be unnecessary.

e False
The woman should be referred to gynaecological outpatients for assessment and D&C.

C22 a True
Meconium may produce gastritis and pylorospasm. If the amniotic fluid is stained with meconium, the newly born infant's stomach should be sucked out to prevent aspiration into the lungs with vomiting. Meconium in the lungs causes aspiration pneumonia.

b True
The abdominal viscera usually occupy the left side of the chest, and displace the heart and mediastinum to the right. If the herniation is large, there may be cyanosis and considerable respiratory distress, exacerbated by pulmonary hypoplasia which co-exists. X-ray will confirm the diagnosis, and emergency surgery should be considered. This condition has now been diagnosed in utero.

c True
Any infection in a baby is likely to present with vomiting. The only other symptoms and signs in meningitis may be a rise in temperature, bulging of the fontanelles and a reluctance to feed.

d False
Necrotising enterocolitis (NEC) typically occurs in a premature infant on SCBU after the first week of life. It can vary in severity from mild with blood and mucus passed per rectum, to severe with shock, perforation, DIC and sloughing of the rectal mucosa. In addition to intensive supportive measures, surgery may be necessary.

e True
Other causes of vomiting in the first 24 hours are: alimentary tract obstruction, e.g. duodenal atresia; feeding mismanagement; cerebral disorders, e.g. intracranial haemorrhage; metabolic and biochemical disorders, e.g. uraemia; and idiopathic.

C23 a True
Fluid restriction may reduce symptoms in these women.

b True
Breast binding is associated with more pain than pharmacological methods in the first week, but appears to be more effective in the longer term.

c True
Bromocriptine inhibits the release of prolactin from the pituitary. For suppression, 2.5 mg is given daily for 3 days and then twice daily for 14 days. It is more effective in the first week post-partum.

d False
Stilboestrol, an oestrogen, does suppress lactation. However, the incidence of side-effects is high. These include abnormal uterine bleeding and thromboembolic disease.

e False
The risk of thromboembolic disease post-partum with the combined oral contraceptive pill is considerable, and therefore its use is contraindicated.

C24 a False
Before birth, the ductus arteriosus carries oxygenated blood into the systemic circulation, bypassing the lungs. With the fall in pulmonary vascular resistance that occurs at birth, there is reversal of blood flow in the ductus arteriosus. It constricts in response to the rise in oxygen pressure in the aortic blood, but remains patent for 2–3 days. It can be kept open longer by giving prostaglandin E_2 in conditions in which this is beneficial, such as transposition of the great vessels. This is a cyanotic form of congenital heart disease that relies on a patent ductus to permit oxygenated blood to reach the systemic circulation.

b True
The ductus venosus allows blood from the umbilical vein to bypass the liver (as the placenta performs most of the functions of the liver before birth). When the umbilical cord is clamped, the venous return from the placenta stops abruptly causing collapse of the ductus venosus.

c False
As the lungs expand and fill with air, the pulmonary vascular resistance falls.

d False
The foramen ovale almost closes functionally as the left atrial pressure rises and the venous pressure drops. A small shunt may persist for 5 days. Anatomical closure does not occur in up to 25% of children.

e True
This must be reduced to a minimum if a drop in infant temperature is to be avoided. The baby should be dried with a warm towel, wrapped in a warm blanket and then held by its parents.

C25 a False
Although it can be suspected antenatally, cephalopelvic disproportion can only be diagnosed in labour and it is rare for a primigravida to be denied a trial of labour. Antenatally, primigravida of less than 155 cm (5′ 1″) in height or with a history of a pelvic fracture should be carefully assessed. However, maternal height and shoe size have been found to have a limited predictive value. Clinical antenatal assessment may include abdominal palpation of the fetal head, vaginal examination and radiological pelvimetry. Warning signs include failure of the cervix to dilate despite the use of oxytocin and, during the second stage, failure of the head to descend to the pelvic floor.

b False
Oxytocin can be used in primigravid women to augment poor uterine contractions, provided the progress of the labour is regularly monitored. Cephalopelvic disproportion can only be diagnosed if there is no progress despite adequate contractions, when abdominal delivery will be indicated.

c False
There is considerable danger of uterine rupture in a parous woman treated with oxytocin. The classical features are a sudden feeling of something giving way, cessation of contractions, hypotension and collapse.

d False
Malnutrition causing pelvic rickets is most uncommon in the UK, but should be considered amongst women of Asian descent.

e False
There must be no cephalo-pelvic disproportion for an instrumental delivery, otherwise there is a significant danger to the mother and fetus.

C26 a True
Spontaneous abortions are significantly increased in diethylstilboestrol exposed women. Otherwise, apart from the risk of premature birth, there are no other consistent unfavourable outcomes. The drug was taken to diminish the risk of spontaneous abortions in the 1940s and 1950s. Other problems include vaginal adenosis and the rare clear cell adenocarcinoma of vagina.

b True
A previous prostaglandin termination may result in uterine synechiae or cervical incompetence. Intra-uterine adhesions predispose to first trimester abortion, while cervical incompetence causes second trimester abortions.

c True
The rate also increases with high gravidity and in lower socioeconomc groups.

d True
The risk is slightly increased in smokers, with the risk of congenital abnormality also increased. Other toxic causes include alcohol, working with anaesthetic gases and radiation.

e False
VDU use is not associated with any harm to pregnant women, and the evidence against VDUs so far is not soundly based. A good review article is: Blackwell et al 1988: Visual display units and pregnancy. British Journal of Obstetrics and Gynaecology 95: 446–453.

C27 a False
Monozygotic twins arise from one ovum that divides. They may be dichorionic diamniotic (separate or fused), monochorionic diamniotic or, more rarely, monochorionic monoamniotic. Monozygotic twins are at risk from twin-to-twin transfusion due to the presence of anastomoses between the two placentas. Dizygotic twins arise from two ova with duplication of the normal process of development. Dizygotic twins have their own membranes (chorion and amnion), placenta and placental circulation, even if the placentas are fused, and so there is no risk of twin-twin transfusion.

b True
Dizygotic twins are more common with increasing maternal age, reaching a peak between 35 and 39 years of age. Other factors causing increased rates include increasing parity, maternal height and nutritional status. Hereditary factors are also important, particularly on the maternal side. Monozygotic twins are more likely to occur as a chance phenomenon.

c True
The incidence of pre-eclampsia is higher in twin pregnancies, and the onset is earlier, particularly in primigravid women. There is probably no difference between monozygotic and dizygotic twins. There is also an increased incidence of polyhydramnios, abortion, pre-term labour and anaemia.

d False
There is no advantage in admitting women with twin pregnancy for bed rest unless there are complications, such as antepartum haemorrhage, pre-eclampsia or threatened pre-term labour. The effect of bed rest on subsequent gestational age is controversial. There are economic and social disadvantages in removing the woman from her family.

e False
The perinatal death rate in twins is 5 times that of singleton neonates. 50% of multiple pregnancies produce low birthweight infants, mainly due to prematurity. Fetal abnormalities are more common. Perinatal loss is greater in the second twin. Growth retardation is also more common in twin pregnancies.

C28 a False
However vitamin D supplements may be required for Asian immigrants to prevent osteomalacia in the mother and rickets and dental enamel hypoplasia in the fetus.

b True
This is often not achieved in the first trimester due to vomiting, but is usually achieved by the second trimester.

c False
There is no need for this, and pregnant women should do what they feel able to do. Later in pregnancy, they inevitably reduce their amount of exercise.

d False
Healthy pregnant women with a good diet need not be given iron routinely. Their haemoglobin should be checked at booking and in the third trimester, and iron prescribed to those who are anaemic.

e False
A woman with a healthy diet does not need vitamin supplements.

C29 a False
The value of this has not been verified. It will produce a great deal of maternal anxiety and a large amount of unnecessary intervention and hospitalisation.

b False
This outmoded examination has no predictive value, and pregnant women dislike vaginal examinations.

c True
This is generally speaking true, but is a poor predictor of performance in labour. A pelvic tumour or low placenta should be excluded by ultrasound examination.

d False
The GP or midwife is capable of these visits and can then refer if necessary.

e False
DOMicilary IN and Out involves the community midwife accompanying her own patient to hospital, delivering her, and then taking her home again after 6 hours. This arrangement, however, is less popular for first labours since the community midwife is committed to one woman for a long time. They are ideal for multiparous women having a short labour.

C30 a False
The perinatal mortality rate is the number of stillbirths and deaths in the first week of life per 1000 total deliveries (still and live). It has fallen in England and Wales, but this fall occurred before the rise in caesarean section rate. Likely factors for this are increased standard of living, reduced parity, screening for fetal abnormality, better maternal services and care, and better neonatal care.

b False
The WHO recommends including all fetuses weighing more than 500 g in perinatal figures. This approximates with 22 weeks gestation. It is not yet in widespread use in the UK.

c False
There are marked regional variations in all countries, which suggests that there are preventable causes. Other factors which increase PNM include: social class (increased in social classes 4 and 5), teenage mothers and mothers over 35, grand multiparity, multiple pregnancy, children of women of Bangladeshi or West Indian extraction, and small-for-dates babies.

d True
The other important causes are hypoxia (18%), placental conditions (16%), birth problems including cord problems (11%), maternal conditions, e.g. pre-eclampsia (8%).

e False
The definition used in the UK is the number of stillbirths and deaths in the first week of life per 1000 total deliveries.

C31 a True
Women presenting with sexual dysfunction in their relationship may be depressed. Skillful and sensitive history taking is required so that the aetiology can be understood. More commonly, the woman will present with depression, and only after direct questioning are the sexual problems exposed.

b True
The tricyclic antidepressants cause dry mucus membranes and may cause dyspareunia. Other drugs, such as alcohol, bendrofluazide and beta-blockers may also cause sexual problems.

c False
Although it may reveal a sexual problem.

d True
This will require sensitive evaluation. If there is not the expertise or resources in the Primary Care Team, referral should be made to a psychosexual counsellor.

e True

C32 a False
Nulliparous women are 3 times more likely to develop endometrial carcinoma than are multiparous women. Risk factors include obesity and the use of oestrogen hormone replacement therapy in postmenopausal women without concurrent progesterone. The link with obesity is via the production of more oestrogen by the peripheral conversion of androgens. Other uncommon causes of high levels of unopposed oestrogens are anovulation associated with the polycystic ovary syndrome, and oestrogen-secreting tumours. In the past, it has been suggested that diabetes mellitus and hypertension are also risk factors, but further studies have not supported this.

b False
It usually presents with postmenopausal bleeding or a watery vaginal discharge. Clinical examination is usually unremarkable. Although cancer cells may be found on a cervical smear, uterine curettage should be performed.

c False
As the incidence of ovarian metastases is 5–10%, bilateral salpingo-oophorectomy should be performed at the time of hysterectomy. An oestrogen implant may be left to prevent menopausal symptoms and osteoporosis.

d True
Medroxyprogesterone acetate 100 mg twice a day may produce a significant response in advanced metastatic endometrial carcinoma. Well-differentiated tumours respond most favourably. It may be useful for women who are considered to be unfit for surgery. Apart from surgery, radiotherapy can be used both pre-operatively and post-operatively.

e False
75% of affected women are postmenopausal, 15% perimenopausal and up to 10% are still menstruating regularly.

C33 a False
Ulceration is an early sign in carcinoma of the vulva, and any ulcerative lesion should be urgently referred for a consultant opinion.

b False
This is never adequate therapy for vulval cancer. The first operation gives the best chance of cure. The main problem with this surgery is delayed wound healing. This can be reduced by performing the operation through separate incisions.

c True
Although not practical due to complications of treating a moist area.

d True
It is uncommon, with about 600 new cases per year. Early disease, however, has a 90% cure rate with appropriate surgery.

e False
It spreads by lymphatics until very late. This accounts for the good survival if the woman presents early.

C34 a False
The highest reported mortality is 18%. Death is usually from starvation. 16% of survivors remain seriously underweight after 8 years. The symptoms of food preoccupation and avoidance, weight loss and amenorrhoea usually start post-puberty at 17 years. 5% will start prepuberty. The female to male ratio is 10:1. The person may induce vomiting and/or use excessive laxatives. If binge eating occurs without weight loss, the term bulimia nervosa is used. Family therapy and admission to specialist units are the most effective therapy for this difficult condition.

b True
Any cause of weight loss of 10 kg or more is frequently associated with amenorrhoea. Serum oestrogen and FSH are low due to reduced hypothalamic-ovarian function. Hormone replacement or ovulation induction is not used unless the woman wishes to become pregnant. Low T3 and blood glucose are found, with raised serum carotene, growth hormone and cortisol.

c True
Up to 10% of female siblings are affected. This may represent a genetic effect, but is more likely to be due to abnormal family dynamics and behaviour.

d False
Avitaminosis is unusual, and most anorexics maintain their vitamin intake.

e False
Breast atrophy does not occur. The physical signs include hypotension, bradycardia and increased lanugo (fine, downy hair growth).

C35 a False
Ovulation occurs approximately 12–24 hours after the LH surge. This is important during IVF, since eggs need to be collected when they are mature but before ovulation. This is therefore done just after the LH surge.

b True
This is the usual method used to confirm ovulation.

c True
This is true however long the cycle is. When pregnancy is being dated from the last menstrual period, it is important to add the number of days by which the cycle exceeds 28 days, e.g. 7 days for a 35-day cycle.

d True
Women should therefore be advised to use contraception if they wish to avoid pregnancy, even if they are still amenorrhoeic from breastfeeding.

e False
This is a pre-ovulatory sign and is used in the Billing's method of natural family planning to indicate to the woman when she is about to ovulate.

C36 a True
The re-absorption of oestrogen is affected by amoxycillin, ampicillin, erythromycin and tetracycline. The gut flora is altered by these antibiotics, and ethinyloestradiol is not deconjugated. As a consequence of less enterohepatic circulation and biliary excretion, more ethinyloestradiol is passed in the stool. Breakthrough bleeding and pregnancy can occur, particularly with low dose oestrogen contraceptive pills. If any of these antibiotics are necessary, the woman should continue to use the pill but should also use a barrier method for the next 14 days. Enzyme-inducing drugs, such as phenytoin, carbamazepine and rifampicin, lower plasma levels of ethinyloestradiol. The pill containing 50 μg of oestrogen should be used in women taking these drugs.

b False

c True

d True

e False

C37 a True
The overall complication rate for vaginal hysterectomy is half that of abdominal hysterectomy. Post-operative fever is the most common complication of both these procedures, but is considerably less in vaginal hysterectomy, providing prophylactic antibiotics are used.

b True
The average age of the menopause is 52 years. The advantage of elective oophorectomy is prevention of the leading cause of cancer mortality in the genital tract in women, particularly as ovarian cancer presents late. Modern hormone replacement protects women against menopausal symptoms and osteoporosis, but does not reproduce the normal hormonal cycle. At present, this does not seem to be a serious disadvantage, but the long-term effects of ovary removal may not yet be fully understood.

c False
Direct ablation of tissue using cryotherapy, electrodiathermy, cold coagulation or laser give high success rates. If the woman does not wish further children, a cone biopsy may be performed. Hysterectomy can be considered if the woman has coexisting benign gynaecological disease.

d True
Although emphasised more by urologists than gynaecologists.

e True
The risk is slightly higher overall for vaginal hysterectomy. The risks increase with age and the presence of coexisting medical conditions.

C38 a True
The commonest sites in the genital tract affected by gonococcus are the endocervix, urethra and, occasionally, the rectum. The gonococcus involves columnar epithelium and so does not affect the stratified squamous epithelium of the vagina as easily. Before puberty, the vaginal epithelium can support the growth of gonococcus, but after puberty only the fornices and cervix are able to do so. *Trichomonas vaginalis* is commonly associated with concurrent gonococcal infection. When a woman presents with an undiagnosed vaginal discharge in general practice, charcoal swabs should be taken from the posterior vaginal fornix, cervix and urethra. A swab using special chlamydial transport medium is also taken from the endocervix. This also allows visualisation of the cervix, and excludes the presence of a foreign body. In practice, as thrush is the most common cause, clotrimazole is the first line treatment.

b True
Bartholin's gland is situated in the posterior third of each labium majus. An abcess forms as a result of infection and blockage of the duct. It is important to differentiate it from an infected sebaceous cyst in the anterior two-thirds of the labium majus, which usually settles with antibiotics. Treatment of an infected Bartholin's cyst should involve a charcoal swab, marsupialisation and penicillin. Occasionally, gonococcus also infects the para-urethral glands (Skene's glands).

c True
Disseminated gonococcal infection is uncommon but women, especially pregnant women, are more often affected. The symptoms range from mild arthralgia to severe destructive arthritis. Gonococcus should always be thought of in a monoarthritis. In 30% of cases, a painful papular or necrotic rash develops. Rare complications include endocarditis and meningitis.

d False
However, it can be transmitted to babies during vaginal delivery, causing ophthalmia neonatorum.

e False
Gonococcal fixation tests are not routine in most laboratories. Laboratory diagnosis is performed by microscopy of Gram stain smears (which show Gram-negative intracellular diplococci), culture and delayed fluorescent antibody staining.

C39 a False
Women with quiescent ulcerative colitis or Crohn's disease at the time of conception have a 50% relapse rate, but this is similar to that in non-pregnant women. The relapses tend to occur in the first trimester and post partum.

b True
Women with Crohn's disease have a significant risk of being infertile, while with ulcerative colitis the evidence is not clear. Salazopyrine, one of the main drug therapies for inflammatory bowel disease, is known to cause male infertility but the effect on women is not known.

c True
Salazopyrine contains a sulphonamide and 5-aminosalicylic acid. Although sulphonamides have the potential to cause palatal and skeletal abnormalities, as well as kernicterus, adverse reports with salazopyrine have so far been few, and it is generally considered safe to use during breastfeeding and pregnancy. It does impair the absorption of folic acid and so supplements of folic acid should be given.

d True
Vitamin B_{12} is absorbed in the terminal ileum and is important in haemopoiesis. If the terminal ileum is diseased, e.g. in Crohn's ileitis, or if it has been resected, supplementary vitamin B_{12} needs to be given. Other elements may be malabsorbed in Crohn's including vitamin D and iron.

e True
Fetal and maternal mortalities are high following surgery, and it is reserved for severe fulminant inflammatory bowel disease. Medical treatment with salazopyrine and corticosteroids is the mainstay of therapy. Metronidazole is commonly used in non-pregnant women, but its safety in pregnancy and breastfeeding has not been proven.

C40 a False
The vaginal diaphragm is more commonly used than the cervical cap. The cervical cap covers the cervix and remains in place by suction. It was originally designed to be worn throughout the menstrual cycle, being removed only at the time of menstruation. However, prolonged use gives rise to vaginal discharge and odour, as well as a risk of developing the toxic shock syndrome. Other problems with the cap are that it must be tailored to fit the cervix exactly, and the cervix changes in size throughout the menstrual cycle. The failure rate is similar to that of the diaphragm. Venules and vault caps are also occasionally used.

b True
All barrier methods protect against cervical neoplasia and sexually transmitted diseases.

c True
After any pregnancy or vaginal surgery, the diaphragm should be checked by a health professional. Changes in weight may also produce changes in the vaginal vault and necessitate alteration in the size of the diaphragm. Otherwise, annual checking of the fit of the diaphragm is sufficient.

d False
The diaphragm (and its covering of spermicidal cream) should not be removed until 6 hours after intercourse. If further intercourse occurs, more spermicidal cream should be introduced into the vagina without removing the diaphragm. One method is to insert the diaphragm at night and then leave it in position until the next evening. The diaphragm is then removed, cleaned and reinserted with new spermicidal cream whether or not intercourse is to occur that evening. The diaphragm is then always in position and its insertion is separate from the act of intercourse.

e False
In motivated women with motivated partners, the failure rate is as low as 3–5 per 100 women years.

7. Paper D

D1 A 28-year-old woman has had three normal deliveries at term of approximately 3 kg babies. In this pregnancy, she is admitted to a GP unit with spontaneous rupture of the membranes at term. Progress to 8 cm is rapid, but three hours later she is still only 8 cm dilated although contracting strongly every 2 minutes. The following statements are true:
   a Intravenous oxytocin should be started
   b Transfer to a consultant unit is indicated
   c Delivery should be expedited using the vacuum extractor (Ventouse)
   d Ultrasound estimation of fetal weight is required
   e Rupture of the uterus is imminent

D2 The following drugs are correctly linked to a recognised side-effect:
   a Methyldopa – pancreatitis
   b Frusemide – haemolytic anaemia
   c Bromocriptine – severe nausea
   d Nitrofurantoin – peripheral neuropathy
   e Phenytoin – gingival hypertrophy

D3 Female sterilisation:
   a Has a higher failure rate if done in the puerperium
   b Causes menorrhagia
   c By laparoscopy, has a mortality of 5 per 100 000
   d Should never be made a condition of termination of pregnancy
   e If it fails, may result in tubal pregnancy

D4   The following are true:
   a Congenital CMV infection may account for 10% of mental retardation by school age
   b 60% of women possess anti-CMV antibodies
   c Carriage of beta haemolytic streptococcus in the vagina is normal
   d There are 2000 cases of congenital toxoplasmosis in the UK per year
   e Toxoplasmosis is a cause of hydrocephalus

D5   A neonate with hepatosplenomegaly may have:
   a Congenital CMV infection
   b Thalassaemia
   c Haemophilia
   d Haemolytic disease of the newborn
   e Trisomy 18

D6   The placenta:
   a Grows throughout pregnancy
   b Has only a small functional reserve
   c Determines fetal growth
   d Secretes HCG throughout pregnancy
   e Secretes oestriol independent of the fetus

D7   Birthweight:
   a Is reduced in babies of teenage mothers
   b Falls with altitude
   c Increases with birth order
   d Increases with increasing maternal weight at booking
   e Is reduced in Asians compared with Caucasians

D8   A 25-year-old woman delivers her second baby (male) weighing 2.9 kg at term (3rd centile). This may be:
   a A normal variation
   b Due to congenital rubella
   c Due to placental insufficiency
   d Due to trisomy 13
   e Due to wrong dates

D9   A pregnancy of 12 days can be diagnosed by:
   a Transvaginal ultrasound
   b Serum beta HCG
   c Pelvic examination
   d Serum progesterone
   e Laparoscopy

D10 Open neural tube defects:
- **a** Are commoner in South Wales than in South England
- **b** Can all be detected using maternal serum alpha fetoprotein
- **c** Can all be diagnosed on real time ultrasound
- **d** The recurrence risk is determined by the presence or absence of other abnormalities
- **e** Are commoner in multiple pregnancies

D11 Down's syndrome (trisomy 21):
- **a** Is better predicted by age and serum alpha fetoprotein than by age alone
- **b** Infants are stillborn in 20% of cases
- **c** Most are born to women under the age of 35
- **d** May be due to a balanced translocation in the father
- **e** Often requires delivery by emergency caesarean section for fetal distress

D12 Respiratory distress syndrome (hyaline membrane disease):
- **a** Tends to be less severe in female neonates
- **b** May be prevented by steroids given to the mother 24 hours prior to delivery
- **c** Is best treated by artificial surfactant
- **d** Occurs in all neonates born before 32 weeks
- **e** May lead to recurrent chest infections in infancy

D13 A pregnant insulin-dependent diabetic:
- **a** Is at increased risk of a fetus with sacral agenesis (caudal regression syndrome)
- **b** May deliver a 4.5 kg baby at term, despite good diabetic control
- **c** Is at increased risk of a baby with a neural tube defect
- **d** Should be delivered by caesarean section
- **e** Increases her insulin requirements by at least 50%

D14 A Bartholin's abscess:
- **a** Is usually treated by incision and drainage
- **b** Occurs on the inner posterior aspect of the labia majora
- **c** May be due to gonorrhoea
- **d** Can be treated by needle aspiration and antibiotics
- **e** If recurs, may require excision of the gland

D15   Which of the following are true?:

a A child conceived by artificial insemination is illegitimate in the UK
b The risk of HIV transmission is reduced if only cryopreserved semen is used
c Oocyte donation has been opposed by the Warnock Committee
d Translaparoscopic gamete intrafallopian transfer (GIFT) requires a patent fallopian tube
e The Roman Catholic Church allows the practice of donor insemination in married couples

D16   Galactorrhoea may be caused by:

a Spironolactone
b Bromocriptine
c Prochlorperazine
d Imipramine
e Metoclopramide

D17   A 26-year-old primigravida is found to have a blood pressure of 160/100 mmHg and 2+ proteinuria at 38 weeks. Which of the following statements are true?:

a She may have a headache and abdominal pain
b Pre-eclampsia is certain
c She should be delivered within 12 hours
d She should be investigated by a renal physician
e She should be given a diuretic

D18   The following recurrence risks are correct:

a One previous open spina bifida   −1%
b One previous pre-term delivery   −30%
c One baby with Down's syndrome   −5%
d One previous caesarean section   −50%
e Pre-eclampsia in a previous pregnancy   −10%

D19   A baby born at 32 weeks is at risk of:

a Bronchopulmonary dysplasia
b Patent ductus arteriosus
c Hypothermia
d Postpartum hypoxia
e Anaemia

D20   An infant born at 42 weeks is at risk of:

a Delivery by caesarean section
b Meconium aspiration
c Erb's palsy
d Transient tachypnoea of the newborn
e Hypoglycaemia

D21 A 24-year-old woman at 8 weeks gestation is in contact with rubella. Which of the following statements are true?:
   a She should be offered vaccination
   b She will be immune if vaccinated as a schoolgirl
   c She can be reassured if rubella serology is negative
   d If she is infected there is a 90% chance of fetal abnormality
   e She should be offered a termination

D22 Oligohydramnios may be associated with:
   a 42 weeks gestation
   b Renal agenesis
   c Tracheo-oesophageal fistula
   d Intra-uterine growth retardation
   e Placenta praevia

D23 Thyroid disease in pregnancy:
   a A goitre usually indicates thyrotoxicosis
   b Raised free T4 indicates thyrotoxicosis
   c Thyrotoxicosis is best treated by surgery
   d Thyroxine does not cross the placenta
   e Carbimazole therapy is a contraindication to breastfeeding

D24 Acute pyelonephritis in pregnancy:
   a Is usually left-sided
   b Rarely causes a fever above 38.5°C
   c Is usually due to Proteus sp.
   d Antibiotic therapy should await urine culture
   e May lead to pre-term delivery

D25 Cardiac disease in pregnancy:
   a Is an indication for termination on medical grounds
   b May be treated surgically to save the mother's life
   c Is an indication for caesarean section
   d Usually requires prophylactic antibiotics for labour and delivery
   e Is a contraindication to syntometrine use in the third stage of labour

D26 Radiotherapy for carcinoma of the cervix may cause:
   a Vesico-vaginal fistula
   b Ovarian failure
   c Ureteric fistula
   d Vaginal stenosis
   e Small bowel obstruction

D27 The fetal skull:

   a The anterior fontanelle is at the junction of the sagittal, frontal and coronal sutures
   b Moulding reduces within 24 hours of birth
   c Moulding is a contraindication to rotational forceps
   d Engages in the submento-bregmatic diameter with a face presentation
   e The mento-vertical diameter is equivalent to the antero-posterior diameter of the pelvic inlet

D28 Mature unexplained stillbirth:

   a Is a rare cause of perinatal death
   b Should be registered
   c Predisposes to thromboembolism
   d Induction is performed by amniotomy and intravenous oxytocin
   e Is non-recurrent

D29 A third degree tear involving the rectal mucosa:

   a Is more likely in women with a narrow sub-pubic arch
   b The incidence is reduced by performing an episiotomy
   c Is more common with vacuum extraction as opposed to forceps delivery
   d Has a small risk of subsequent recto-vaginal fistula, even if repaired immediately by an experienced operator
   e Is sutured following infiltration of local anaesthetic

D30 The uterus is supported by:

   a The broad ligament
   b The uterosacral ligaments
   c The transverse cervical ligament
   d The falciform ligament
   e The round ligament

D31 Women originating from the Indian subcontinent have an increased rate of:

   a Cephalopelvic disproportion
   b Babies dying in the perinatal period
   c Babies with congenital malformation
   d Babies who die of sudden infant death syndrome
   e Anaemia

D32 Genital infection with Herpes simplex:

   a May cause acute retention of urine
   b Is a cause of carcinoma of the cervix
   c Acyclovir therapy reduces the time of viral shedding
   d The virus persists in the sensory neurones
   e Caesarean section is only required for primary infection at the time of delivery

D33 Disseminated intravascular coagulation is commonly caused by:
 a Uterine rupture
 b Abruptio placentae
 c Placenta praevia
 d Amniotic fluid embolism
 e Gram-negative septicaemia

D34 Useful methods of assessing fetal well-being in the third trimester include:
 a Serum oestriol estimation
 b Ultrasound assessment of amniotic fluid volume
 c Serum alphafetoprotein estimation
 d Fetal breathing
 e Fetal tone

D35 Sickle cell disease:
 a Is commoner in Africans than West Indians
 b For two homozygous parents (HbAS), the chance of an affected child is 1 in 4
 c Is a preventable cause of death in the first year
 d Is an indication for pneumococcal vaccination
 e In pregnancy, will require regular blood transfusions

D36 Regarding skin disorders in the first month:
 a Cavernous haemangiomas (strawberry naevus) will usually fade
 b Infantile eczema will have manifested itself
 c Granuloma annulare may indicate systemic disease
 d Miliaria rubra is due to photosensitisation
 e Mongolian blue spots are associated with Down's syndrome

D37 The following agents are suitable for long-term prophylaxis against urinary tract infection in pregnancy:
 a Ampicillin
 b Nitrofurantoin
 c Co-trimoxazole
 d Erythromycin
 e Nalidixic acid

D38 The following are recognised problems with artificial feeding:
 a Jaundice
 b Obesity
 c Tetany
 d Vitamin deficiency
 e Diarrhoea

D39 Cystic fibrosis:
a Is amenable to population screening of carriers
b Failure to thrive is due to recurrent chest infections
c Prenatal diagnosis may not be possible if there is no genetic material from living relatives available
d Regular physiotherapy is necessary
e The high sweat sodium may lead to rapid dehydration in hot weather

D40 The following conditions are associated with pregnancy:
a Carpal tunnel syndrome
b Meralgia paraesthetica
c Facial nerve palsy
d Common peroneal nerve palsy
e Acute infective polyneuropathy (Guillain-Barré syndrome)

8. Paper D Answers

D1 **a False**
Oxytocin should be administered to multiparous women with great care and only in a consultant unit.

b True
Transfer is required.

c False
Although the use of the Ventouse has been described before full dilatation, it is potentially dangerous for both mother and baby. A caesarean section is the safest method of delivery in this situation.

d False
An estimation of the fetal weight is of no clinical use in this situation.

e True
Urgent caesarean section is required, as rupture of the uterus is the likely outcome. A multiparous woman should have achieved a vaginal delivery by now.

D2 **a False**
Side-effects of methyldopa include sedation at the beginning of therapy, postural hypotension, positive Coombs' test, haemolytic anaemia and, more rarely, abnormal liver function and jaundice.

b False
Haemolytic anaemia is not a recognised side-effect of frusemide. Pancreatitis is a rare side-effect of frusemide but may be more common in pregnancy. Diuretics are only indicated for heart failure in pregnancy, and should not be used to treat oedema as this is a normal response to pregnancy.

c True
This can be a troublesome side-effect, as it is the only treatment for hyperprolactinaemia.

d True
Nitrofurantoin is a useful chemotherapeutic agent and can be used in pregnancy. Peripheral neuropathy is rare, and more likely if there is renal impairment or anaemia.

e True
This is a relatively harmless side-effect, but more serious ones include bone marrow depression, drug rash and congenital hydantoin syndrome (a group of fetal abnormalities associated with phenytoin use in the first trimester). Cardiac arrhythmias can occur with parenteral use.

D3 a True
The true failure rates of different methods of sterilisation are difficult to ascertain. The generally quoted failure rate of interval sterilisation is 2 per 1000. It may be up to 10 times higher if done in the puerperium, and other complications are also increased since a mini-laparotomy is required.

b False
There is no conclusive data to support this. Heavy periods may be revealed once the contraceptive pill is stopped, but this does not mean it is due to the sterilisation.

c True
It must not be forgotten that the (usually) social operation of female sterilisation is potentially fatal. Vasectomy, because it is done under local anaesthetic, is likely to be safer.

d True
This is never the time to consider sterilisation. If the woman is already awaiting sterilisation then it can be performed at the same time, but the complication rate may be higher.

e True
This is true whatever method of sterilisation is used.

D4 a True
CMV infection is asymptomatic or causes a non-specific illness, and is the commonest viral infection in pregnancy. Screening has not been shown to be useful and a vaccine is not available.

b True
This means that 40% of the pregnant population is susceptible. Infection can lead to miscarriage, stillbirth, hydrocephalus, mental retardation, deafness and blindness.

c True
It is common, and population screening in pregnancy is neither effective, practical nor advisable. Swabs should be taken, however, if the membranes rupture pre-term, and conservative management is instituted.

d False
There are approximately 400 births of babies with congenital toxoplasmosis, although it is possible that the incidence is increasing. It is acquired from cat faeces or from eating raw meat.

e True
Congenital toxoplasmosis can cause microcephaly, cerebral
calcification, hydrocephaly and mental retardation, amongst other
things. Treatment of the pregnant woman may reduce the fetal
damage.

D5 a True
This is one of the manifestations of congenital infection.

b True
Babies with thalassaemia have a persistent preponderance of HbF
and a deficiency of HbA. Haemolysis thus occurs and massive
hepatosplenomegaly results.

c False
Haemophilia is a clotting disorder and does not lead to haemolysis
or hepatosplenomegaly.

d True
Haemolytic disease can be due to rhesus or ABO incompatibility.
With the widespread use of anti-D, many cases of haemolysis are
due to antibodies against antigens other than D.

e True
Cardiac abnormalities in trisomy 18 may cause heart failure which
leads to hepatosplenomegaly.

D6 a True
New villi are formed up to term, and there is capacity for
compensating hypertrophy.

b False
The placenta has a large functional reserve, since up to 30% of villi
can be rendered functionless by perivillous fibrin deposition
without the fetus being compromised.

c False
Fetal growth is not determined by placental size. The small placenta
is a manifestation, not a cause, of poor fetal growth.

d True
HCG is secreted by the syncytiotrophoblast even before
implantation. The level peaks at 14 weeks, drops by 18 weeks and
then is secreted at a steady level.

e False
The secretion of oestriol is dependent on the feto-placental unit.
Separately, they lack vital enzymes but they function together in
steroidogenesis.

D7 a True
Teenage mothers tend to have smaller babies than women in their
twenties. This may be a social class phenomenon.

b True
This is due to the reduction in the partial pressure of oxygen in the
atmosphere.

c True
Birthweight rises from first to second and, to a lesser degree, from second to third pregnancy. This may be related to increased maternal weight and a better physiological response to pregnancy.

d True
It also increases with maternal height.

e True
The mean birthweight for Caucasians is 300 g lower *higher* than for Asians (3200 vs 2900 g).

D8 a True
Birthweight follows a normal distribution curve, and a weight on the 3rd centile (−2 Standard Deviations) could be normal, particularly if the woman's last baby was of similar size. Fetal weight is not synonymous with fetal growth, and it is not always possible to know if a baby has fulfilled its growth potential. Thus, a baby destined for the 60th centile (for weight) that only reaches the 20th centile is growth retarded.

b True
Congenital infection is a cause of small-for-dates babies. This term is preferred to growth retardation since it is easier to define.

c True
This is unlikely in a parous woman, unless she has a new partner or had placental insufficiency in her last pregnancy.

d True
Congenital abnormality is another cause of a small-for-dates baby.

e True
This could be eliminated if an ultrasound examination had been performed between 16–22 weeks gestation. This can predict delivery within 5 days even more accurately than can certain dates.

D9 a False
Transvaginal ultrasound should be able to diagnose an intra-uterine pregnancy at approximately 28 days after conception, by the presence of a gestational sac. A fetal node and fetal heart would not be detected for another week. These figures are approximately one week ahead of abdominal scanning.

b True
Beta HCG estimations are highly sensitive and can confirm pregnancy from 10 days onwards. Urinary HCG assays are now almost as sensitive.

c False
The earliest one could suspect pregnancy by pelvic examination would be 8 weeks, and this would need to be confirmed by a pregnancy test.

d True *false*
Although the serum progesterone does rise in pregnancy, it is not sensitive or specific enough to be of diagnostic use.

e False
Neither an intra-uterine nor an ectopic pregnancy would be seen at this early stage. This is a significant problem, since the HCG will be positive 2–3 weeks before a sac can be seen on ultrasound. Therefore, a positive pregnancy test and an empty uterus is not diagnostic of an ectopic pregnancy at very early gestations.

D10 a True
There is a well-recognised geographic variation in the incidence of neural tube defects. The highest incidence is in South Wales and Northern Ireland, and the lowest in South East England.

b False
Any screening test has a false-negative rate and this depends on the cut-off value used and the incidence of the disease. A cut-off at 2.5 multiples of the median for that population will detect 80% of fetuses with open spina bifida, but identify 3% of normal pregnancies.

c False
The accuracy of real time ultrasound as a screening technique (as opposed to its use with a known raised maternal serum AFP) has not been fully evaluated. Reports from specialised units cannot be extrapolated to general use and, since ultrasound is almost entirely operator-dependent, cases will inevitably be missed.

d True
The recurrence risk for an isolated spina bifida is 1 in 20 (5%). If it is part of a syndrome, then the recurrence risk is likely to be lower.

e True
Multiple pregnancy is a cause of a raised serum alpha fetoprotein but, since congenital abnormalities are common in multiple pregnancies, detailed ultrasound examination is required.

D11 a True
Screening for Down's syndrome can be performed using maternal serum AFP and, in itself, will add no extra cost to those units already offering MSAFP for neural tube defect screening. There may, however, be a rise in the rate of amniocentesis. The prediction can be further refined using serum oestriol and hCG.

b True
Hence, careful examination of all stillbirths is required, including cytogenetics of the baby or placenta.

c True
Although the risk is greater in women over 35, most births occur to younger women who therefore have most of the Down's syndrome babies. This is the reason behind the recent interest in screening the whole population.

d True
The parents of a baby with Down's should have their chromosomes checked. If a balanced translocation is present, the recurrence risk depends on the type and, in rare types, can be 100%.

e True
Abnormal babies do not tolerate labour well and are often delivered for fetal distress.

D12 a True
The reason for this clinical observation is unclear.

b True
Maternal administration of steroids between 28 and 32 weeks has been shown to be effective in reducing the incidence and severity of respiratory distress syndrome. The same may be true at earlier gestations, and the benefit of the steroids appears to last up to 7 days.

c True
The use of artificial surfactant reduces morbidity and mortality. The optimum dosage and duration of therapy has not yet been fully established.

d False
Although most infants of this gestation will show some evidence of respiratory distress syndrome, it is by no means universal. Babies which were under some form of 'stress' in utero, e.g. severe pre-eclampsia, seem to need less respiratory support.

e True
This is particularly true of infants requiring prolonged periods of ventilation. It may be that some of the local protective mechanisms have been damaged.

D13 a True
The rate of congenital malformations is quoted as being up to 4 times that in non-diabetics. This may be reduced by very tight control in the first trimester. Caudal regression syndrome is almost totally confined to diabetics.

b True
Approximately 10% of the population will deliver babies of this size, and if the baby is genetically destined to be this size, only placental insufficiency from any cause (e.g. pre-eclampsia) will prevent it. Although good diabetic control will reduce perinatal mortality, it is not as effective at reducing the incidence of macrosomia as was once thought.

c True
Screening with maternal serum AFP must be interpreted with caution, since diabetic women tend to have lower values and hence a lower cut-off should be used.

d False
Vaginal delivery can often be safely achieved, although the caesarean section rate for diabetics will be higher than average, at around 30%.

e True
Pregnant women have a lower sensitivity to insulin and so normally will secrete more endogenous insulin. In a diabetic, the requirements will thus increase from early pregnancy.

D14 a False
Marsupialisation is the technique of choice and involves excising an ellipse of vaginal skin and abscess wall. This allows much better drainage, and reduces the incidence of recurrence.

b True
This is the anatomical position of Bartholin's gland.

c True
A sample of pus should thus be sent for culture, since treatment with penicillin would then be required. Antibiotics are not otherwise indicated.

d True
Recently, there have been reports of this method with a fair amount of success. It will obviate the need for a general anaesthetic.

e True
This is best avoided if possible, since it is a difficult procedure and the scar can lead to dyspareunia.

D15 a True
However, the English Law Commission and the Warnock Committee have recommended that the law is reformed, so that there is no legal distinction between legitimate and illegitimate children.

b True
This allows regular serum testing for HIV in the donor. Cryopreserved semen is preserved for 3 months and should only be used if the repeat HIV test is negative. However, cryopreserved semen has a lower success rate than fresh semen.

c False
It is a recognised technique, and subject to the same regulations as donor insemination, including anonymity of the donor and limitation to 10 of the number of children born from the oocytes of one woman.

d True
Oocytes are recovered laparoscopically and transferred immediately with prepared semen into the end of the fallopian tube. It therefore requires a patent tube to be present, and is mainly used for idiopathic infertility, minimum endometriosis or where there are male factors.

e False
Artificial insemination is rejected for married as much as for
unmarried couples in the Roman Catholic Church. Orthodox
Judaism and the Anglican Church also disapprove of the practice.

D16 a False
This drug is known to cause gynaecomastia in men, which
disappears on stopping the drug. Its main side-effects are
hyperkalaemia and hyponatraemia.
b False
This is the drug of choice for hyperprolactinaemia, a common
cause of galactorrhoea.
c True
All phenothiazines are recognised causes of hyperprolactinaemia.
d True
Tricyclic antidepressants can cause hyperprolactinaemia.
e True
Other drugs known to cause hyperprolactinaemia include digoxin
and reserpine.

D17 a True
If these symptoms are present they indicate fulminating disease
and delivery must be expedited.
b True
By definition, this woman has pre-eclampsia. It is still possible that
she has an underlying cause, such as chronic renal disease, but in
these cases they tend to present early. Phaeochromocytoma as a
cause can present at any gestation.
c False
If she is asymptomatic, then a strict time limit such as this is
unnecessary. In practice, with severe pre-eclampsia at this
gestation the cervix is often favourable and induction easy.
d False
It would be too early to make a judgement on the need for referral
for further investigation. If either the hypertension or proteinuria
had not settled by 3 months after delivery, then referral to a
physician would be indicated.
e False
Diuretics are contraindicated in established pre-eclampsia, since
the intravascular volume is already depleted. Any further depletion
may precipitate renal failure.

D18 a False
The recurrence risk is 1 in 20, i.e. 5%, although it may be lower if
other abnormalities had also been present. Vitamin supplements
are usually prescribed in any future pregnancy.

b False
The risk of a second pre-term delivery is 15%. This means that the chance of a term delivery is almost 7 to 1. Any proposed treatment, e.g. cervical suture, is therefore highly likely to succeed! Furthermore, many of these pre-term deliveries will occur after 34 weeks when the morbidity and mortality are relatively low.

c False
The recurrence risk for most chromosomal abnormalities is 1%. It is considerably higher if either parent has a balanced translocation.

d True
In the UK, approximately 50% of women with a previous caesarean section will undergo a repeat operation in the next pregnancy. This is considerably lower if the reason for the first section was non-recurrent, e.g. breech presentation. In the USA, more than 85% of women with one caesarean section undergo a repeat operation.

e True
The disease tends to be less severe on a subsequent occasion, but not always. It may be preventable by low dose aspirin.

D19 a True
This is particularly so if the baby requires ventilation for prolonged periods. It is not a common sequelae at 32 weeks, and is more common with very low birthweight babies (less than 1000 g).

b True
This is characterised by a loud continuous murmur which is diagnostic. It can lead to heart failure and pulmonary hypertension. Treatment with indomethacin may be successful, but if not, surgery is required.

c True
Pre-term babies easily become cold, and care should be taken to keep them warm.

d True
This may be caused by unrecognised respiratory distress syndrome.

e True
This tends to occur at 2 to 3 months of age. It is probably due to a disparity between intake and the rapid rate of growth at this age. Occasionally, it occurs earlier due to (temporary) marrow hypoplasia.

D20 a True
Caesarean section is commoner at 42 weeks than at 40 weeks for both dystocia and fetal distress.

b True

The incidence of meconium staining of the liquor increases with gestational age. There is evidence that aspiration can occur in utero rather than at delivery, and it is commoner in an asphyxiated fetus. A paediatrician should be present at delivery when meconium has been seen.

c True

Erb's palsy is the result of a brachial plexus injury. This can be caused by excessive traction on the neck if shoulder dystocia occurs. This is commoner at 42 weeks.

d True

This condition occurs particularly after caesarean section. It may be that lung fluid has not been expelled, as occurs during a vaginal delivery.

e False

This occurs more commonly in pre-term infants. It may also occur in infants of diabetic mothers.

D21 a False

Although it has not been clearly shown to be dangerous, it is generally advised that pregnant women are not given vaccinations. It is more prudent to immunise women against rubella before they contemplate pregnancy.

b False

Immunity to rubella following vaccination is not always lifelong, and immunity should be checked at booking.

c False

As with any viral infection, it takes 10–14 days for the antibody response to be detected. If she is not immune on the first blood test, it must be repeated after 14 days.

d True

In the first trimester maternal rubella almost invariably leads to fetal infection, whereas in the second and third the risk is much lower.

e False

Such action is only to be recommended if infection is confirmed. Most women will be immune and, providing this is confirmed, no further action is required.

D22 a True

Oligohydramnios (deepest pool less than 3 cm) is a recognised problem with post-dates pregnancies. It may represent some decline in placental function and induction should be considered.

b True

One constituent of amniotic fluid is fetal urine and hence if not produced oligohydramnios will result.

c False
This will lead to polyhydramnios, because the fetus cannot swallow the liquor and the normal circulation of amniotic fluid is obstructed.

d True
If there is placental insufficiency then amniotic fluid production is low. Similarly, the fetal kidneys do not produce normal amounts of urine.

e False
There is no alteration in amniotic fluid production with placenta praevia.

D23 a False
Although this may be the case, thyroid function tests are likely to be normal. Many goitres of pregnancy are due to a low-iodine diet leading to thyroid hyperplasia to maintain production of thyroid hormones. Iodine is now added to salt and so goitre is rare.

b True
This test is now routinely available, as opposed to thyroid binding globulin (TBG) which is raised in pregnancy anyway.

c False
Thyrotoxicosis can usually be treated in pregnancy using carbimazole or propylthiouracil. Surgery need only be considered in the rare instances when this fails, or a large goitre causes obstruction.

d False
Therefore, babies of mothers with thyroid disease should be closely monitored in the neonatal period.

e True
Carbimazole is excreted in breast milk and, hence, therapy is a contraindication to breastfeeding.

D24 a False
Pyelonephritis affects the right kidney more often and this is thought to be due to the degree of pregnancy-induced renal tract dilatation being more marked on the right.

b False
Pyrexia of 40°C is not uncommon, and is associated with rigors.

c False
Escherischia coli is the commonest cause of urinary tract infection. Organisms such as *Proteus* tend to occur with instrumentation, catheterisation and prolonged antibiotic use.

d False
These women are very ill, and therapy must not be withheld. Culture can take at least 48 hours. Intravenous ampicillin would be a reasonable first line drug.

e True
Any severe infection may lead to pre-term delivery.

D25 a False

Most cardiac conditions are compatible with a relatively good outcome. With the sharp reduction in rheumatic heart disease, congenital heart disease is as common. The only instance where the risk of pregnancy is high enough to warrant termination is Eisenmenger's syndrome (reverse left-to-right shunt).

b True

Conditions such as severe aortic stenosis or incompetence may need to be surgically treated, and the mother's life takes precedence. The fetus may in fact survive surgery anyway.

c False

Most women with cardiac disease will labour well. Induction is not usually needed except for obstetric reasons. Epidurals can be used, but hypotension must be avoided.

d True

Any condition for which there is a risk of endocarditis should be covered by intravenous antibiotic prophylaxis.

e True

Ergometrine is best avoided, because it can cause marked elevation in blood pressure.

D26 a True

This is a well-recognised complication but it is less common with modern megavoltage therapy. It tends to occur late, i.e. minimum 6 months post treatment.

b True

This is an inevitable consequence of pelvic irradiation, and is the reason surgery is preferred for early disease in young women so that the ovaries can be conserved. Hormone replacement therapy can be given.

c False

This is an early complication of surgery, but with an experienced surgeon and no pre-operative irradiation the incidence should be no more than 1%.

d True

This, along with the problem of ovarian failure, is a common cause of dyspareunia. Topical oestrogen and vaginal dilators are used in the treatment of this problem.

e True

This is a very late complication (years) and follows stricture formation. Surgery can be difficult, because multiple areas of bowel may be affected.

D27 a True

This is the position of the anterior fontanelle, and is usually felt in an occipito-posterior position. The posterior fontanelle is at the junction of the lambdoidal and sagittal sutures, and will be felt in a well-flexed occipito-anterior position.

b True

Moulding is a normal phenomenon during which the parietal bones slide under each other, and the occipital and frontal bones under the parietal bones. It rapidly disappears after delivery.

c False

Some degree of moulding is normal and cannot be a contraindication to a safe vaginal delivery. It can be graded, however, and if it is severe it would indicate rotational forceps delivery to be unwise.

d True

The submento-bregmatic diameter is 9.5 cm. This is the same as the presenting diameter in a flexed vertex presentation (sub-occipito-bregmatic). Hence, face presentations usually deliver spontaneously.

e False

This is the presenting diameter in a brow presentation and is equal to 13 cm. The normal antero-posterior diameter of the pelvic inlet is 12 cm. Most brow presentations will convert spontaneously to a face or vertex presentation. If they do not, caesarean section will be required.

D28 a False

This category now accounts for up to 90% of stillbirths. These figures remain the biggest challenge to modern antenatal care.

b True

Any baby born dead after 28 weeks is legally bound to be registered. The parents should be asked if a post-mortem can be carried out, since other causes may be uncovered.

c False

There is no link with thromboembolism. Disseminated intravascular coagulation may occur if the baby has been dead for at least 3 weeks.

d False

The membranes should be left intact for as long as possible as the risk of intra-uterine infection is high. Induction is thus usually performed using vaginal prostaglandins.

e False

There remains a recurrence risk, albeit small. Careful supervision is required and induction may be prudent around 38 weeks.

D29 a True

In this situation, the head is forced posteriorly to find space, and more extensive perineal damage is likely. It may also occur with a rapid uncontrolled delivery.

b False

For spontaneous vaginal deliveries, the data available show an equal incidence of third degree tear whether an episiotomy is performed or not. The prevention of a third degree tear does not in itself appear to be a reason to perform an episiotomy.

c False

Randomised studies have consistently shown a higher rate of third degree tears with forceps.

d True

It is estimated that this may occur in up to 1% of third degree tears, even if sutured by an experienced operator. Most of these fistulae are small and will heal spontaneously.

e False

They should be sutured in optimal conditions. This means in a room with good light and either a regional block or general anaesthetic.

D30 a False

This does not give any support to the uterus. It carries blood vessels, lymphatics and nerves, and is simply a fold of peritoneum.

b True

This is one of the main supporting structures of the uterus. It is used to support the vault after prolapse operations.

c True

This is the other main support of the uterus.

d False

The falciform ligament is attached between the liver and the anterior abdominal wall.

e False

The round ligament does not support the uterus.

D31 a True

This may partly be due to British obstetric practice and perhaps because the women living in the UK have bigger babies than they would in their country of origin. The mean birthweight of their babies remains lower than for Caucasian babies.

b True

Some of this excess is due to congenital malformation and some due to social and environmental factors.

c True
The incidence of lethal malformations is twice that for Caucasians. This is particularly so for autosomal recessive conditions consequent on consanguinous marriages. However, not all of this increase is due to genetic factors, as malformations are also commoner in Hindu and Sikh communities which do not have a large number of such marriages.

d False
The incidence of sudden infant death syndrome (SIDS) is at least half that of white babies.

e True
This is due to many factors such as nutritional deficiencies, thalassaemia trait and pregnancies close together.

D32 a True
Primary infection with Herpes simplex is characterised by the appearance of vesicles which rapidly rupture, forming shallow ulcers which coalesce. These ulcers are exquisitely painful, and retention of urine is a result of this pain. It may be exacerbated by a sacral radiculomyelitis. Treatment is by supra-pubic catheterisation until the lesions crust over and the pain subsides (10–12 days).

b False
Although there is a higher prevalence of antibodies to Herpes simplex in the sera of women with cervical carcinoma, viral DNA has not been demonstrated in cervical cancer cells. The association simply implies exposure to sexually transmitted diseases.

c True
Acyclovir is an expensive drug which inhibits DNA synthesis. In primary infections, intravenous therapy reduces the time for healing, the rate of new lesion formation and the time of viral shedding. Its use in recrudescent lesions is less impressive.

d True
The reactivated virus passes to a peripheral site and a lesion develops. Patients undergoing recrudescence of herpes have (temporarily) impaired T-cell immunity.

e True False
Neonatal herpes is a rare but very serious condition. If primary infection occurs at the time of delivery 40% of babies will develop it if delivered vaginally. The risk is reduced, although not eliminated, by caesarean section before the membranes rupture. In the cases of recrudescent lesions maternal HSV antibody will cross the placenta and protect against generalised disease. It will not protect against localised infection to the eyes and skin and hence caesarean section is still advisable.

D33 a False

Uterine rupture in itself is not associated with DIC. It is, however, a cause of shock and blood loss and massive blood transfusion can be associated with clotting factor deficiency.

b True

This condition is classically associated with disseminated intravascular coagulation (DIC). The degree correlates with the degree of placental separation, although this degree is often difficult to judge clinically. The DIC is initiated by thromboplastin release from the decidua at the separation site. The condition will not resolve until the uterus is empty.

c False

Placenta praevia can cause massive blood loss. With a large blood transfusion, some degree of clotting disorder can occur if the clotting factors are not also replaced in sufficient quantity as fresh frozen plasma (FFP).

d True

This is another well-recognised cause of DIC. It is such a rapidly progressive disorder that the maternal mortality remains very high. Treatment aims to support the circulation, maintain oxygenation by ventilation and replace the clotting factors. Anticoagulation with heparin may prevent further intravascular coagulation and break the cycle of continuing consumption of clotting factors.

e True

Gram-negative bacterial infections can trigger DIC. Treatment must be directed at the cause, as the DIC will not stop until the factors that initiated it have been removed.

D34 a False

Oestriol estimations have not been used in clinical practice for 5 years or more. They are a very insensitive measure of fetal well-being and cannot indicate with any great accuracy when a fetus should be delivered.

b True

A normal liquor volume is a good clinical sign which can be measured on ultrasound examination. Oligohydramnios results from underproduction by the placenta and the fetal kidneys.

c False

Raised serum alpha fetoprotein is a risk factor for third trimester problems, such as small-for-dates babies. However its sensitivity is too low to be of clinical use.

d True

The presence of fetal breathing movements is a healthy sign. It may however be necessary to scan for at least 30 minutes before it can be said to be absent. Its absence may also indicate that labour is about to start.

e False
Although this is part of the Biophysical Profile, it is of little use on its own and is the most subjective part of the score. Furthermore, it is given an equal score to that of liquor volume and CTG reactivity, whereas in practice they are not all equally sensitive.

D35 a True
This may be an evolutionary phenomenon since it protects against malaria, which is not found in the Caribbean.

b True
It is an autosomal recessive condition and hence this is the risk for EACH pregnancy. Pregnant women of Afro-Caribbean origin should be offered screening, as should their partners.

c True
If the condition is unrecognised, a fatal sickling crisis could occur. Prevention by regular blood transfusions and early antibiotic therapy for infections will significantly reduce infant mortality and morbidity.

d True
Pneumococcal pneumonia and meningitis are much commoner in people with sickle cell disease, and they should be offered vaccination.

e True
Regular transfusions will maintain a high proportion of circulating HbA and reduce the stimulus to erythropoiesis so that production of further sickle cells is reduced. This will thus reduce the likelihood of sickling disease during the pregnancy which may result in miscarriage, stillbirth or pre-term delivery.

D36 a True
These are soft, raised red lesions which do not usually appear until some days after birth. They initially enlarge during the first 6 months. Most have disappeared by 7 years, so that surgery is reserved for the few that do not. In general, spontaneous regression does not leave a noticeable scar, whereas treatment often does.

b False
This usually takes up to 3 months to manifest. The severity fluctuates but frequently resolves by puberty. Treatment should be taught to parents, and mainly revolves around the frequent use of emulsifying ointments. Steroids should only be used for very severe episodes.

c False
This condition is characterised by small, firm papules or nodules in a circle or semi-circle. They usually remit spontaneously.

d False
It is a heat rash and occurs due to blockage of sweat ducts. It is another condition which remits spontaneously.

e False
These blue spots are commonly seen over the sacrum and buttocks
and look like bruises. They are only found in infants of Oriental or
Afro-Caribbean origin, and fade during infancy. They have no
association with Down's syndrome.

D37 a False
Ampicillin is not suitable for long-term prophylaxis, as resistant
strains are inevitable and may be very difficult to eradicate.

b True
It is associated with very rare side-effects of peripheral neuropathy
and haemolysis in the neonate. This latter condition is more likely
in infants with glucose-6-phosphate dehydrogenase deficiency.
Nitrofurantoin passes into the breast milk.

c False
Co-trimoxazole is not suitable for use in pregnancy because of its
anti-folate action.

d False
Erythromycin is not a drug used in the treatment or prophylaxis of
urinary tract infection.

e True
This is not an antibiotic, but concentrates in the urine and is a useful
drug in this context. It does not cross the placenta.

D38 a False
This is not a specific complication of bottle feeding. Mean serum
bilirubin levels, however, are lower in breast-fed babies.

b True
The old idea of 'fat babies being healthy babies' has been dispelled.
Fat babies are overfed, but it is difficult to overfeed a breast-fed
baby.

c True
Newborn infants with tetany develop focal myoclonic jerks,
sometimes followed by generalised fits and cyanosis. Cow's milk
has a lower calcium/phosphate ratio than breast milk, and hence
serum calcium levels are lower in bottle-fed babies.

d False
Artificial feeds are fortified with vitamins. Vitamin D and K and iron
deficiency can easily occur in breast-fed babies, and supplements
need to be given.

e True
This is probably due to excess sugar or fat in bottle-fed babies. True
cow's milk allergy is uncommon. Breast-fed babies rarely get
diarrhoea, although their stools may seem very loose to an
inexperienced mother.

D39 a True
1 in 25 of the population carries the cystic fibrosis gene and about one child in every 2000 has the disease. It is now possible to identify these carriers by a mouth wash which sheds enough cells from the buccal mucosa. This is much more acceptable for population screening than a blood test.

b False
Pancreatic insufficiency plays a major role but is now amenable to treatment with artificial enzymes.

c True
The exact locus of the cystic fibrosis gene has not been found and therefore genetic material from affected and non-affected members of the same family is required to compare with genetic material from the fetus.

d True
This is a major part of the treatment of an affected child, and the parents need to learn to give it themselves.

e True
Care must be taken to ensure that this does not happen.

D40 a True
The median nerve passes between the flexor retinaculum and the bones of the wrist. This space can become compressed in pregnancy by the generalised oedema. Carpal tunnel syndrome can be a very distressing condition, and if it does not respond to splinting and hydrocortisone injections surgical decompression may be required.

b True
The pathophysiology of meralgia paraesthetica is the same as the carpal tunnel syndrome, but it affects the lateral cutaneous nerve of the thigh as it passes over the iliac crest. Treatment is less successful, but the condition will resolve after pregnancy.

c True
Facial nerve palsy is commoner in the third trimester of pregnancy than at any other time. The facial nerve passes through a long bony canal as it leaves the skull, and can become compressed by the oedema of pregnancy. The condition slowly resolves after delivery.

d True
Some cases of pregnancy-related foot drop will be due to pressure from the use of lithotomy poles. Cases can occur following normal delivery due to compression of the cords of L4 and L5 as they pass into the pelvis.

e False
This is a rare condition that follows a generalised viral infection. It is no more common during pregnancy.

9. Paper E

E1 Active management of the third stage of labour:

a Reduces the incidence of postpartum haemorrhage
b Increases the incidence of retained placenta
c Reduces the length of the third stage to a mean of 5 minutes
d Is less effective with an epidural in situ
e Involves giving 0.5 mg ergometrine with the anterior shoulder

E2 Causes of primary amenorrhoea include:

a Cryptomenorrhoea
b Turner's syndrome
c Polycystic ovary syndrome
d Lawrence-Moon-Biedl syndrome
e Testicular feminisation

E3 Acute retention of urine in women may be due to:

a Primary genital herpes
b Multiple sclerosis
c Ectopic ureter
d An ovarian cyst the size of a 20-week pregnancy
e Posterior colpoperineorrhaphy

E4 The following features are common to both endometriosis and chronic pelvic inflammatory disease:

a Deep dyspareunia
b Secondary dysmenorrhoea
c Fixed retroversion of the uterus
d Nodules on the uterosacral ligaments
e Menorrhagia

E5 Impending eclampsia is heralded by:

a Occipital headache
b Photophobia
c Epigastric pain
d Rising urate levels
e Fetal tachycardia

E6 Infection with *Listeria monocytogenes*:
a Causes mid-trimester miscarriage
b May present as pyelonephritis
c Causes meningitis in the neonate
d Is confirmed by culture of a high vaginal swab
e Is treated by doxycycline

E7 Pre-term rupture of the membranes at 30 weeks gestation is associated with:
a Painful contractions
b Breech presentation
c An abnormal fetus
d Chorioamnionitis
e Urinary tract infection

E8 A normal 6-week infant:
a Plays with his/her hands
b Has a positive Moro reflex
c Will only follow objects less than 12 inches away
d Will have had his/her first immunisation
e Has head control

E9 Malignant disease of the vulva is associated with:
a Atypical hyperplastic dystrophy
b Genital herpes infection
c Genital warts
d Lichen sclerosus
e Carcinoma of the cervix

E10 Progestogen-only pills:
a Have no thromboembolic risk
b Increase the risk of ectopic pregnancy
c Inhibit ovulation
d Make the cervical mucus more viscous
e Cause irregular menstruation

E11 Vulvo-vaginitis in an 8-year-old girl may be due to:
a Poor hygiene
b A foreign body
c Sexual abuse
d *Candida albicans*
e Threadworms

E12 Normal labour in a primigravida:
a Cannot be diagnosed until the cervix is at least 3 cm dilated
b Amniotomy may be useful
c The fetus should be continuously electronically monitored
d Requires oxytocin in approximately 30% of cases
e Is slowed by epidural analgesia

E13 Toxic shock syndrome:
a Is due to toxins from gram-negative coliforms
b Causes a rash, high fever and renal failure
c Is strongly associated with the use of super absorbent tampons
d Is treated with high dose penicillin
e Has a mortality of 50%

E14 Concerning trisomy 18 (Edward's syndrome):
a The incidence is increased in women over 35 years of age
b Cleft lip and palate are a feature
c The diagnosis can be suspected by the ultrasound appearance of the skull
d Affected infants are usually male
e Caesarean section is often necessary for fetal distress

E15 Postmenopausal bleeding may be due to:
a Urethral caruncle
b CIN 3
c Carcinoma of the fallopian tube
d Atrophic vaginitis
e Stress

E16 The following organisms can be detected on a cervical smear:
a *Candida albicans*
b *Actinomyces israeli*
c *Herpes simplex*
d *Trichomonas vaginalis*
e Human papilloma virus (HPV)

E17 Measurement of serum FSH and LH:
a Can confirm the occurrence of the menopause
b Levels of both are low in anorexia nervosa
c Can be used to diagnose polycystic ovary syndrome (PCO)
d Should be performed on day 12 of the cycle in the investigation of subfertility
e Levels are normally reduced for three months after stopping the oral contraceptive pill

E18 Hyperprolactinaemia:
a May be due to the use of metoclopramide
b Occurs in response to stress
c Inhibits ovulation
d Is associated with hypothyroidism
e When due to pituitary microadenoma always responds to bromocriptine

E19 The following are true:

 a All births must be registered within 48 hours
 b A baby born alive at 24 weeks who dies after 10 minutes does not need to be registered
 c A stillbirth at 28 weeks gestation weighing less than 500 g is not included in perinatal mortality statistics
 d The death certificate for a stillborn baby can be signed by a registered midwife
 e Neonatal deaths are required to have a post-mortem

E20 Osteoporosis:

 a May be caused by long-term steroid use
 b After the menopause, is due to poor calcium intake
 c Is more effectively prevented by oestradiol implants than oral oestrogen
 d Has no diagnostic test
 e Is irreversible

E21 Polycystic ovary syndrome:

 a Can be diagnosed by ultrasound
 b Should be treated with the oral contraceptive pill if pregnancy is not desired
 c Causes relative oestrogen deficiency
 d Is associated with an increased risk of endometrial carcinoma
 e Is resistant to clomiphene

E22 Genital warts:

 a Can cause koilocytes on a cervical smear
 b Grow during pregnancy and regress after delivery
 c Are associated with carcinoma of the vulva
 d Local treatment with podophyllin can cause peripheral neuropathy due to systemic absorption
 e Are an indication for yearly cervical smears

E23 Detrusor instability can be successfully treated by:

 a Biofeedback
 b Flavoxate HCl (Urispas)
 c Terodolin
 d HRT if postmenopausal
 e Bladder distension

E24 The following drugs cross the placenta:

 a Metronidazole
 b Labetalol
 c Heparin
 d Chlormethiazole
 e Diazepam

E25 Inversion of the uterus:
a Is largely prevented by active management of the third stage of labour
b Produces profound shock
c Bleeding is usually minimal
d Is non-recurrent
e May be due to a morbidly adherent placenta

E26 The following increase the risk of carcinoma of the endometrium:
a An early menopause
b Maturity onset diabetes
c High parity
d Atypical endometrial hyperplasia
e Obesity

E27 The following statements concerning treatment of carcinoma of the ovary are true:
a The prognosis depends on the amount of tumour remaining at the end of the first operation
b Stage 1a tumours require a 6-month course of methotrexate
c A second look laparotomy is required at 6 months
d Radiotherapy is effective
e Unilateral salpingo-oophorectomy is adequate for early stage dysgerminomas in young women

E28 The use of antenatal corticosteroids in pre-term labour:
a Reduces the severity of respiratory distress syndrome
b Reduces the severity of periventricular haemorrhage
c Increases the severity of neonatal hypoglycaemia
d Reduces the severity of necrotising enterocolitis
e Increases the severity of neonatal sepsis

E29 Pulmonary embolism:
a Haemoptysis is the commonest symptom
b Characteristically occurs 5 days after delivery
c Breastfeeding should be interrupted if an isotope lung scan is performed
d Heparin overdose can be treated with prostigmine
e May occur antenatally

E30 The following are a contraindication to a further attempt at vaginal delivery after a previous caesarean section:
a Postpartum sepsis
b A vertical incision on the uterus
c Extended breech presentation
d Cephalopelvic disproportion
e Bicornuate uterus

E31 The following are recognised side-effects of Danazol:
a Hirsutism
b Weight loss
c Decreased serum HDL and cholesterol
d Hot flushes
e Peripheral oedema

E32 Placenta praevia:
a Causes 10% of third trimester antepartum haemorrhages
b Can be overdiagnosed on ultrasound if the bladder is empty
c Is associated with transverse lie
d Typically causes severe pain and bleeding
e Has an increased incidence following previous caesarean section

E33 A pregnant woman of Afro-Caribbean origin:
a Is more likely to smoke cigarettes
b Characteristically has an android pelvis
c Is more likely to be delivered by caesarean section
d Delivers babies of smaller average birthweight than Caucasian women
e Is more likely to breastfeed

E34 Which of the following statements concerning the female pelvis are true?:
a The sub-pubic angle is more acute than in the male
b The pelvic cavity is deeper than in the male pelvis
c All diameters of the mid-cavity are approximately 12 cm
d The bony pelvis is the most important factor in determining whether a woman will achieve a normal delivery
e The pelvic outlet is bounded by the lower part of the pubis anteriorly and the coccyx posteriorly

E35 Urge incontinence:
a Is best treated by a colposuspension operation
b May be an early symptom of multiple sclerosis
c Is always due to detrusor instability
d May be helped by vaginal oestrogen cream
e Is a rare condition

E36 Which of the following statements concerning the Apgar score at 5 minutes are true?:
a A heart rate of 100 bpm scores 1
b A pink body and blue extremities scores 2
c Some limb flexion scores 1
d Vigorous crying in response to stimulation scores 2
e Irregular breathing scores 2

E37 The vaginal contraceptive sponge:
  a Uses the spermicidal, nonoxyl-9
  b Has a failure rate similar to the combined contraceptive pill
  c Is contraindicated in a woman who has previously suffered from the toxic shock syndrome (TSS)
  d Can be used during menstruation according to the manufacturers' instructions
  e Requires fitting by a health professional

E38 With which of the following symptoms or signs is it safe to discharge a woman from hospital following a laparoscopic sterilisation?:
  a Shoulder tip pain
  b Mild vaginal bleeding
  c Abdominal tenderness
  d Hypotension
  e Impaired consciousness level following a general anaesthetic

E39 Which of the following are absolute contraindications to an epidural in labour?:
  a Refusal by the woman
  b Sepsis in the lumbosacral area
  c Maternal coagulopathy
  d Low dose heparin
  e Past history of back pain

E40 Napkin rash in an infant of 6 weeks is likely to be due to:
  a Seborrhoeic dermatitis
  b Eczema
  c Intertrigo
  d Candidiasis
  e Ammoniacal dermatitis

10. Paper E Answers

E1 **a True**
The benefits of routine administration of oxytocics and controlled cord traction for the third stage of labour have been clearly shown.

b True
Although the increase is small in comparison with the marked reduction in postpartum haemorrhage. The main problem is that an anaesthetic is required.

c True
A passively managed third stage can last 20 minutes or longer.

d False
An epidural has no influence on the third stage.

e False
In most units, a combination of 5 units oxytocin and 0.5 mg ergometrine is given intramuscularly (1 ampoule of Syntometrine). Oxytocin alone should be used for women who are hypertensive or have cardiac disease.

E2 **a True**
This is due to a blockage to the outflow of menstrual blood and is usually caused by an imperforate hymen. It is easily treated by incising the membrane.

b True
The diagnosis has sometimes been made before puberty and withdrawal bleeding will occur with hormone replacement. Many cases present with primary amenorrhoea as the only symptom.

c False
Polycystic ovarian disease usually presents with irregular periods, anovulation and hirsutism.

d True
This is due to a rare hypothalamic-pituitary disturbance and will have been diagnosed in childhood (mental retardation, retinitis pigmentosa and polydactyly).

e True
Although genetically male, these patients are female in all other ways and should be treated as such. The testes are usually in the inguinal canal and should be removed to prevent malignant change.

E3 a True
Primary infection with genital herpes is very painful and often made worse by secondary bacterial infection. The resulting acute retention is best relieved by supra-pubic catheterisation.

b True
Retention of urine (other than after surgery or childbirth) is very rare, and neurological causes must be excluded. In practice, multiple sclerosis more commonly causes urinary frequency.

c False
This causes incontinence because it usually opens below the bladder neck in women.

d False
A cyst of this size would not impact on the pelvis and hence will not cause retention. It is likely to cause frequency and a feeling of incomplete emptying.

e True
A common complication of vaginal surgery. Supra-pubic catheterisation is often preferred post-operatively because it avoids repeated catheterisation.

E4 a True
This is due to scarring, infiltration of the utero-sacral ligaments and adhesions that pull the ovaries into the pouch of Douglas.

b True
Although these are classic causes of secondary dysmenorrhoea, in practice most cases are not due to either of these conditions.

c True
Again, due to chronic scarring.

d False
This is diagnostic of endometriosis (c.f. **a**).

e True
Although these are both recognised causes of menorrhagia, most cases are due to dysfunctional uterine bleeding.

E5 a False
Frontal headache is a characteristic feature of impending eclampsia, although other causes of headache may need to be considered (e.g. migraine).

b True
Women with suspected pre-eclampsia should have fundoscopy to exclude the presence of papilloedema.

c True
Epigastric pain is a serious symptom in pre-eclamptic women and is due to liver oedema and stretching of the capsule.

d False
Although this may be a feature of worsening pre-eclampsia, it is not related to the risk of eclampsia. Women can be seriously ill with pre-eclampsia and never have a fit. Urate levels are used to assess the degree of renal impairment in pre-eclampsia, and levels have been shown to correlate with perinatal outcome.

e False
There is no correlation with the fetal heart rate.

E6 a True
It is an uncommon cause of miscarriage but is potentially preventable. Listeria contaminates soft cheeses, unpasteurised milk and, more recently, some 'cook-chill' foods.

b True
A non-specific febrile illness and loin pain are early features.

c True
It therefore has a high mortality unless recognised and treated early.

d False
Blood cultures are required to make the diagnosis.

e False
High-dose ampicillin is the treatment of choice.

E7 a True
Pre-term labour and delivery occur within a week in most cases of pre-term rupture of the membranes.

b True
Premature babies account for 25% of babies born by the breech. Delivery is often by caesarean section if the baby is considered viable and believed to weigh less than 1.5 kg.

c True
Abnormal babies often deliver prematurely.

d True
Once this has occurred, delivery must be expedited for maternal and fetal reasons. Antibiotics should be started.

e False
However, genital tract infection may have an aetiological role. Whether this is cause or effect is uncertain.

E8 a False
They may begin to find their hands by this age, but don't generally start to play with them for another few weeks.

b True
This would be present until about 3 months of age. Sudden movement of the neck initiates rapid abduction and extension of the arms and opening of the hands. The arms then come together.

c True
Infants of this age can follow objects very close to their face that move from side to side. Their eyes do not show focusing and convergence until 8 weeks.

d False
The new schedule starts diphtheria, tetanus and polio at 8 weeks, but there is evidence that immunisation can begin soon after birth.

e False
Some minor degree of support is exhibited, but not proper head control. Head lag on pulling to a sitting from a lying position is normal.

E9 a True
There are many types of vulval dystrophy and the classification has recently been modified. Any evidence of cellular atypia increases the risk of subsequent carcinoma, and careful follow-up is required.

b False
This has no link with subsequent malignant change.

c True
Although warts are common and carcinoma rare, there is a well-recognised association.

d False
There is no association between lichen sclerosus and vulval carcinoma.

e True
Whether the wart virus is the link remains uncertain, but women with carcinoma of the cervix have an increased risk of developing carcinoma of the vulva later.

E10 a True
Progestogens are not linked to venous thrombosis. They are, however, linked with arterial disease (including hypertension). Newer progestogens, e.g. desogestrol, may have a lower risk.

b True
The risk is small and probably due to an effect on tubal motility.

c False
Although this may occur, the mechanism of its contraceptive action is its effect on the endometrium and cervical mucus.

d True
This makes it much more difficult for spermatozoa to penetrate the mucus.

e True
This remains the main disadvantage of this form of contraception.

E11 a True
Advice regarding hygiene and frequent bathing will be needed.

b True

A general anaesthetic may be required for a full examination of a girl of this age.

c True

A careful history from both the child and her mother is required. An examination looking for stigmata of sexual abuse will be required, and this should preferably be performed by someone with training and experience in child abuse.

d True

Lack of protective oestrogen leads to a lowered acidity in the vagina. This means the vulva and vagina are more easily infected by opportunist organisms.

e True

This follows peri-anal itching and scratching.

E12 a False

Labour is diagnosed when regular painful contractions lead to effacement and progressive dilatation of the cervix. This may be accompanied by a show or rupture of the membranes. If, on admission, the cervix is effaced and 1 cm dilated, and two hours later is 3 cm dilated, a diagnosis of labour can confidently be made. The use of terms such as 'early labour', 'not in established labour' or 'latent phase' are not generally helpful.

b True

Whether it should be done as a 'routine' is debatable, but there is little doubt that it speeds up a slow labour.

c False

There may be benefits of continuous electronic fetal monitoring for slow labours and those requiring oxytocin. It has not been shown to improve the outcome in labours lasting less than 5 hours.

d True

If a partogram is used with a view to labour not lasting more than 12 hours, then oxytocin augmentation will be required in about 30% of first labours. Because of this level of intervention, booking primigravidas for delivery in isolated GP units is unwise.

e False

The length of the second stage may be prolonged due to a lack of bearing down, but epidurals do not prolong the length of labour.

E13 a False

Exotoxins from *Staphylococcus aureus* are the cause of the toxic shock syndrome.

b True

Hence, a gynaecological cause for such symptoms may not be thought of initially.

c True
Although cases unrelated to menstruation may have been recorded, most are associated with the use of super-absorbent tampons. They are widely available in the USA, where most cases have been reported, but not on sale in the UK. The syndrome can occur with all types of tampons and does occur in the UK.

d False
High dose flucloxacillin is required as *Staphylococcus aureus* is invariably resistant to penicillin. Broad-spectrum antibiotics will be required if secondary superinfection occurs.

e False
The mortality is approximately 5%.

E14 a True
All trisomies are commoner in women over the age of 35.

b False
This is a feature of trisomy 13.

c True
Apart from the characteristic skull shape, other features may be recognised on ultrasound, e.g. hypoplastic lungs, rocker-bottom feet, cardiac abnormalities and exomphalos.

d False
They are invariably female. Male fetuses probably abort spontaneously.

e True
Abnormal babies tolerate labour badly, and if the abnormality is unrecognised caesarean section will be performed.

E15 a True
This may be considered as the cause once a diagnostic curettage has excluded an endometrial cause.

b False
Cervical intra-epithelial neoplasia is asymptomatic.

c True
A rare condition which is very difficult to diagnose. Recurrent postmenopausal bleeding for no apparent cause may raise suspicion.

d True
This is the commonest cause. Diagnostic curettage is still required.

e False
Postmenopausal bleeding must never be explained away by stress or anxiety.

E16 a True
If asymptomatic, may not need treatment as it may be a commensal.

b True
Particularly in a wearer of a plastic intra-uterine contraceptive device (Lippes' loop). It may occasionally occur with copper devices. Treatment with penicillin is usually only required if the woman is symptomatic.

c False
The virus can only be 'seen' by electron microscopy. Laboratory diagnosis is usually by immunofluorescence or DNA analysis.

d True
Treatment with metronidazole is required.

e False
Evidence of HPV infection may be manifest by the presence of koilocytes. These cells show vacuolation due to the cytopathic effect of the virus.

E17 a True
Levels over 40 i.u. for both LH and FSH are diagnostic of ovarian failure.

b True
Oestrogen levels are also low.

c True
An LH:FSH ratio of 3:1 or more on day 2 of the cycle is regarded as diagnostic of PCO.

d False
An LH surge prior to ovulation would give a falsely raised result.

e False
Post-pill amenorrhoea is no longer regarded as a clinical entity. Hyperprolactinaemia and premature ovarian failure will be missed if amenorrhoea is put down simply to the contraceptive pill.

E18 a True
Metoclopramide and all phenothiazines are well-recognised causes of a raised serum prolactin. Other drugs causing hyperprolactinaemia include haloperidol, methyldopa, imipramine and cimetidine.

b True
Even the anxiety of having the blood taken can raise the level of prolactin.

c True
Ovulation usually returns with appropriate treatment.

d True
Other causes include sarcoidosis, chronic renal failure, craniopharyngiomas and TB meningitis.

e True
If response does not occur, the diagnosis should be questioned. A macroadenoma or Cushing's disease may be present.

E19 a False
All births are notified immediately, but registration is allowed up to 6 weeks after.

b False
It is a neonatal death and requires registration and a death certificate. This applies to any fetus born alive.

c False
This baby must be registered and given a death certificate.

d True
A registered midwife can sign a death certificate for a stillborn baby.

e False
A post-mortem can only be arranged without parental consent on the orders of a coroner.

E20 a True
Osteoporosis is a reduction of bone mass and particularly affects the axial skeleton. As well as the menopause, prolonged immobility and steroid use are common causes.

b False
It is due to lack of oestrogens.

c False
There is no good evidence to show an advantage of one route of administration over another.

d False
Standard X-ray and radio-nuclide scanning can be used for diagnosis but not screening. Bone densitometry by two interval scans can be used for screening but is too expensive for widespread use.

e True
Although bone density may be marginally improved by treatment, previous architectural bone strength cannot be achieved and the fracture rate remains high. Prevention is possible with oestrogen, but the question remains whether all women should be treated or whether it is possible to identify an at-risk population.

E21 a False
High-resolution ultrasound can identify enlarged ovaries with a thickened cortex and multiple cysts. However, this does not always correlate with any biochemical abnormalities characteristic of the syndrome.

b False
Treatment is indicated for cycle control or contraception, as spontaneous ovulation can occur. However, there is concern that chronically low oestrogen levels associated with anovulation may lead to osteoporosis. It is not clear whether this risk is real enough to recommend treatment for all women with PCO.

c False
Women with PCO have high circulating levels of oestrone as well as luteinising hormone, testosterone and androstenedione. They have low levels of sex hormone binding globulin.

d True
This is due to prolonged exposure to oestrogen (albeit low levels) without any protective progesterone. This may be another reason to suggest treatment for all women with PCO.

e False
This condition characteristically responds well to stimulation, although the pregnancy rate is not as high as one would expect.

E22 a True
Koilocytes are cells showing vacuolation due to the cytopathic effect of HPV.

b True
Unless causing severe symptoms, treatment is best deferred until after delivery since it is then much easier. The woman should be screened for other sexually transmitted diseases.

c True
However, warts are common and cancer of the vulva rare. Other factors obviously play a part.

d True
This treatment has a low success rate, whereas treatment with the laser or diathermy is very effective. These methods require a general anaesthetic.

e False
Although HPV may have a role in the aetiology of cervical carcinoma, the time from infection to development of the disease will remain long. Several working parties have recommended screening no more than every 3 years.

E23 a True
This technique is time-consuming but very effective (80% reported success). The relapse rate, however, is also about 80%.

b False
This has not been shown to be of use.

c True
This is the drug treatment of choice. As well as being anti-cholinergic, it is a calcium channel blocker. The side-effects of dry mouth and blurred vision are less marked than other anti-cholinergic agents.

d True
A very effective treatment.

e False
This may have a short-term placebo effect but is not widely used.

E24 a True
This drug should therefore be avoided in the first trimester, although specific fetal effects have not been described.

b True
It thus affects the fetal heart and the fetal response to glucose, which may be important if delivery follows.

c False
Heparin is the anti-coagulant of choice in the first trimester. Warfarin does cross the placenta and is teratogenic in the first trimester.

d True
Chlormethiazole may cause neonatal respiratory depression. It is also excreted in breast milk, and its use has been superseded by diazepam or, more recently, phenytoin.

e True
It can therefore cause neonatal hypotonia and respiratory depression in the neonate.

E25 a True
Only a relaxed uterus can undergo inversion and, hence, the use of oxytocics will protect against inversion.

b True
The shock may be out of proportion to the blood loss, possibly due to excessive vagal stimulation.

c False
Blood loss is usually significant.

d False

e True

E26 a False
A late menopause is a risk factor, possibly due to a longer exposure to endogenous oestrogens.

b True

c False
Parous women have a lower risk of endometrial and ovarian cancer.

d True
This carries an estimated 20% risk of endometrial cancer and hence hysterectomy is indicated. Simple cystic hyperplasia can be treated with cyclical progestogens, and has a less than 1% risk of developing into carcinoma.

e True
Oestrogen is produced in adipose tissue and hence obese women may have relatively high levels. Needless to say, other factors must also be involved.

E27 a True
Whether this is a reflection on the surgeon or the tumour remains
unclear. The first operation should remove as much tumour as
possible and, in order to maximally debulk ovarian cancer, bowel
resection may be required.

b False
This has been shown to be unnecessary and runs the risk of causing
a second tumour, i.e. leukaemia.

c False
This does not in itself confer a survival advantage and there is at
present no effective second line treatment if a full course of
chemotherapy has been given.

d False
It may have a role as an adjuvant in stage 1c disease, but ovarian
tumours (except dysgerminomas) are more susceptible to
chemotherapy than to radiotherapy.

e True
Several successful pregnancies have been reported after treatment
for early stage dysgerminoma. Pelvic clearance is usually
recommended once their family is complete.

E28 a True
It therefore follows that morbidity and mortality are reduced by
antenatal steroids given to the mother.

b True

c False
This is a theoretical risk which has not been shown in practice.

d True

e False
(c.f. **a**.)

E29 a False
Haemoptysis is not very common. Chest pain and shortness of
breath are more common symptoms.

b False
Day 10–14 is the classical time for a pulmonary embolus. The risk is
increased over the age of 35, after caesarean section and by obesity.

c True
The isotope used is rapidly excreted from the body, so
breastfeeding need only be interrupted temporarily.

d False
Protamine sulphate can be given, but the half-life of heparin is so
short that protamine is rarely required.

e True
Risk factors include previous thromboembolism and pre-
eclampsia, particularly with prolonged bed rest.

E30 a False
This is often quoted as a reason to deny subsequent attempts at vaginal delivery, but there is no published evidence to support it.

b True
Any vertical incision on the uterus may lead to rupture, even prior to labour. It appears that transverse incisions are only liable to rupture in labour.

c False
An extended breech presentation is not an absolute contraindication, and vaginal delivery can be anticipated in most cases.

d False
50% of women who undergo caesarean delivery for 'dystocia/failure to progress/cephalo-pelvic disproportion' can subsequently deliver vaginally, often of bigger babies.

e False
Although the incidence of malpresentations is higher.

E31 a True
Danazol is a synthetic androgen. It is indicated for the treatment of endometriosis, benign breast diseases (e.g. fibrocystic mastitis), menorrhagia and the premenstrual syndrome. Other side-effects include acne, vaginal bleeding, hot flushes, voice changes, decreased breast size and atrophic vaginitis.

b False
A small weight gain is common, and reflects increased anabolic activity. Increases greater than 4 kg (10 lb) are not common, but are associated with higher doses and prolonged treatment.

c True
HDL and cholesterol fall with danazol and return following stopping the drug. This is one of the reasons for restricting the length of use. It should not be used for women known to be hyperlipidaemic.

d True
This is due to the anti-oestrogen effects of danazol.

e True
This may make the treatment unacceptable to many women. However, none of these side-effects is long-term, and they are reversible on stopping the drug.

E32 a True

b False
An over-distended bladder can produce a false appearance of placenta praevia by compressing the lower uterine walls together and increasing the apparent length of the cervix.

c True
Since it prevents a presenting part entering the pelvis.

d False
Is classically a painless bleed.

e True
The risk is approximately 3%. Other risks include multiparity and increasing age.

E33 a False
These women are less likely to smoke cigarettes. They may, however, consume other drugs such as cannabis and cocaine which also have documented adverse effects on pregnancy.

b True
The African pelvis is characteristically android, and the inlet resembles a triangle in shape rather than an oval. It also has a high angle of inclination and the head does not engage in the pelvis until very late in the first stage, or even the second stage, of labour.

c True
Dysfunctional labour is commoner in Afro-Caribbean women and, even if an active approach is undertaken, the rate of primary caesarean section is higher than for Caucasians.

d True
This is largely genetic, and appropriate growth and weight charts need to be constructed for different racial groups.

e True
These women are more likely to breastfeed, and for longer.

E34 a False
The sub-pubic angle is less acute in the typical female pelvis. In the android type of pelvis, it is more acute and thus forces the fetal head posteriorly.

b False
The male pelvis has a deeper pelvic cavity.

c True

d False
The efficiency of the uterine contractions is the most important factor.

e False
The outlet is bound by the last fixed point of the sacrum. The coccyx is not considered suitable as it is so mobile.

E35 a False
Operative measures for urge incontinence are not generally helpful. The management depends on the cause. Urinary tract infection, bladder tumour etc. need appropriate treatment. Detrusor (the muscle of the bladder wall) instability is best treated by anticholinergics such as terodiline (Terolin 12.5–25 mg twice a day) or tricyclic antidepressants. Unfortunately, it is often unresponsive to treatment.

b True
Detrusor hyper-reflexia may result from upper motor neurone
lesions, such as spinal cord injury, multiple sclerosis and CNS
tumours. Therefore, women who present with these symptoms
should have at least a brief neurological examination, especially of
the lower limbs.

c False
Other causes include those in **a** and **b**, as well as radiation cystitis,
bladder stones, bladder outflow obstruction and lack of oestrogen
in postmenopausal women.

d True
After excluding a urinary tract infection, the GP can try local
hormone replacement cream in postmenopausal women. This
treatment will reduce symptoms in a significant number of women.

e False
Among women over 18 years of age, pure stress incontinence
occurs in 9% and combined stress and urge incontinence in 14%.
The urge component increases with the woman's age.

E36 a False
The Apgar score is as shown below:

Sign	Score		
	0	1	2
Heart rate	Absent	Under 100/min	Over 100/min
Respiratory effort	Absent	Weak, irregular	Strong, regular
Muscle tone	Limp	Some limb flexion	Active movement
Reflex irritability	No response	Cry	Vigorous cry
Colour	Blue, pale	Body pink, limbs blue	Completely pink

It is measured at 1 and 5 minutes. The key features are the heart rate
and the respiratory effort. It is a useful scoring system, but has
limitations. Other criteria, such as the time taken to first gasp or to
establish regular respiration, may be more useful. As previously
stated in this book, the Apgar score may be a measure of fetal
asphyxia but is a poor predictor of subsequent cerebral palsy.

b False
This situation scores 1.

c True

d True

e False
Irregular breathing scores 1.

E37 a True
Therefore no additional spermicidal cream is used. This method is less messy than conventional barrier methods. It works as a barrier, as a carrier of spermicide and as a sponge to absorb semen.

b False
The sponge has higher failure rates than the combined oral contraceptive pill or the diaphragm with spermicidal cream. It should therefore not be used in young women in whom pregnancy is undesirable. It is more appropriately used in women aged over 44 until 1 year after the menopause, and in lactating mothers.

c True
There is a slightly increased incidence of the toxic shock syndrome (TSS) in sponge users. Some doctors do not advise using the sponge during menstruation. If the woman has had previous TSS, the sponge is contraindicated.

d True
Although medical opinion suggests that the sponge may cause TSS particularly if used during menstruation, the manufacturers still advise it may be used during menstruation but it must be removed 6 hours after intercourse.

e False
It is designed to be bought over the counter without a prescription. The woman inserts it after moistening it with tap water. No special fitting is required. It can be inserted up to 24 hours prior to intercourse and offers protection for 24 hours. It is removed by means of a tape at least 6 hours after the last sexual contact. It is not felt by the male. It has a very high acceptability but is expensive.

E38 a True
Shoulder tip pain is common. The carbon dioxide introduced during the procedure may irritate the diaphragm and cause referred pain in the shoulder as both have the same sensory nerve supply. The woman should be given adequate analgesia but can be discharged.

b True
A D&C of the uterus is often carried out initially during the procedure. A rigid instrument is then introduced into the uterine cavity so that it can be manoeuvred during the laparoscopy. Some mild vaginal bleeding is common, but if the loss is heavy or increasing the woman should remain in hospital and be examined to look for a cause.

c False
Women with abdominal tenderness should be fully assessed. The carbon dioxide can cause tenderness, particularly if it has not been released at the end of the procedure. Other causes, such as bowel injury, vascular injury and mesosalpinx injury, may require further operative measures. If such symptoms occur, the woman is best observed until they settle or a cause is determined.

d False

The cause of the hypotension must be found and treated. If the woman is shocked, blood should be sent for crossmatching and she should be resuscitated. After resuscitation, laparotomy may be required to ascertain the cause.

e False

The woman should fully recover before she is discharged. She should not drive and must be escorted home by a sensible adult. She should be advised to report back to the hospital or to her GP if she experiences problems.

E39 a True

b True

Sepsis in this region is rare. An epidural needle should not be introduced, especially if the needle passes through the infected area.

c True

Certain conditions predispose to coagulopathy, e.g. pre-eclampsia and placental abruption. It is essential that coagulation studies are done in at-risk groups immediately before the epidural.

d False

Anticoagulation other than low dose heparin is an absolute contraindication. Women on low dose heparin should have their coagulation checked.

e False

It is a relative contraindication on medico-legal grounds. Any woman with a chronic neurological or back condition could be assessed by a senior anaesthetist in the third trimester, and epidural discussed. It is important to document any such discussions in the notes in case a relapse occurs following the epidural.

E40 a True

This is a transient, non-itchy rash seen in infants under 3 months. It affects the scalp (cradle cap), the axillae, the flexures and the trunk. It usually resolves without treatment, but can be helped by 1% hydrocortisone cream.

b False

This is uncommon in infants under 3 months and is associated with a family history of atopy. Treatment involves using 1% hydrocortisone cream and emulsifying ointment instead of soap.

c True

It results from rubbing of skin surfaces together. Fat babies are particularly prone to it. Treatment involves keeping the area dry by using dusting powders, avoiding plastic pants, and other measures that reduce sweating.

d True
Candidiasis is particularly common. Satellite lesions around the main rash are typical. Oral thrush should be looked for. Treatment with topical nystatin, clotrimazole or miconazole together with oral nystatin suspension is effective.

e True
Ammoniacal dermatitis results from infrequent nappy changes and may result from neglect. It only affects the skin in the nappy area and does not affect the flexures. The best treatment is leaving the nappies off for 1–2 days. Zinc and castor oil cream will help clear it up.

Recommended Reading

WORTH BUYING

Enkin M, Keirse M, Chalmers I 1989 A guide to effective care in pregnancy and childbirth. Oxford University Press, Oxford
Guillebaud J 1986 Contraception. Your questions. Churchill Livingstone, Edinburgh
Kaye P 1988 Notes for the DRCOG. Churchill Livingstone, Edinburgh
Liu D, Lachelin G 1989 Practical gynaecology. Butterworths, London
Rymer J et al 1990 Preparation and revision for the DRCOG. Churchill Livingstone, Edinburgh
Vulliamy D G, Johnston P G B 1987 The newborn child, 6th edn. Churchill Livingstone, Edinburgh

OTHER BOOKS WITH USEFUL CHAPTERS

Collier J, Longmore J 1989 Oxford handbook of clinical specialities. Oxford University Press, Oxford
de Sweit M 1989 Medical disorders in obstetric practice, 2nd edn. Blackwell Scientific, Oxford/London
Stirrat G M 1983 Aids to obstetrics and gynaecology for MRCOG Part 2, 2nd edn. Churchill Livingstone, Edinburgh
Studd J 1990 Progress in obstetrics and gynaecology, 7th edn. Churchill Livingstone, Edinburgh
Symonds E M 1987 Essential obstetrics and gynaecology. Churchill Livingstone, Edinburgh
Turnbull A C, Chamberlain G V P 1989 Obstetrics. Churchill Livingstone, Edinburgh

Index

The questions have been indexed under either gynaecology, neonatology or obstetrics. The letter and number refer to the question paper and the number on the paper respectively. (The number in brackets refers to the page number.)